Comparative Effectiveness Research

Comparative Effectiveness Research

Mary A. M. Rogers

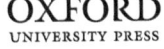

OXFORD
UNIVERSITY PRESS

Oxford University Press is a department of the University of Oxford.
It furthers the University's objective of excellence in research, scholarship,
and education by publishing worldwide.

Oxford   New York
Auckland   Cape Town   Dar es Salaam   Hong Kong   Karachi
Kuala Lumpur   Madrid   Melbourne   Mexico City   Nairobi
New Delhi   Shanghai   Taipei   Toronto

With offices in
Argentina   Austria   Brazil   Chile   Czech Republic   France   Greece
Guatemala   Hungary   Italy   Japan   Poland   Portugal   Singapore
South Korea   Switzerland   Thailand   Turkey   Ukraine   Vietnam

Oxford is a registered trademark of Oxford University Press
in the UK and certain other countries.

Published in the United States of America by
Oxford University Press
198 Madison Avenue, New York, NY 10016

© Oxford University Press 2014

All rights reserved. No part of this publication may be reproduced, stored in a
retrieval system, or transmitted, in any form or by any means, without the prior
permission in writing of Oxford University Press, or as expressly permitted by law,
by license, or under terms agreed with the appropriate reproduction rights organization.
Inquiries concerning reproduction outside the scope of the above should be sent to the Rights
Department, Oxford University Press, at the address above.

You must not circulate this work in any other form
and you must impose this same condition on any acquirer.

Library of Congress Cataloging-in-Publication Data
Rogers, Mary A. M., author.
Comparative effectiveness research / Mary A.M. Rogers.
   p. ; cm.
Includes bibliographical references.
ISBN 978-0-19-998604-0 (alk. paper)
I. Title.
[DNLM: 1. Comparative Effectiveness Research—methods.   2. Data Collection—methods.
3. Evaluation Studies as Topic.   4. Research Design. W 84.3]
R853.C55
610.72′4—dc23
2013029710

To my mother, DeLellis

CONTENTS

About the Author   ix

1. The Reason   1
2. The Question   10
3. The Choice   19
4. The Effect   43
5. The Design   60
6. The Person   121
7. The Place   135
8. The Time   141
9. The Fit   149
10. The Plan   166
11. The Inspiration   182

Bibliography   189
Index   197

ABOUT THE AUTHOR

Mary A. M. Rogers, PhD, MS, is a Clinical Epidemiologist who received her degree at the University of Washington in Seattle. She began teaching integrated science in the Peace Corps and has spent her career teaching and conducting clinical research. Dr. Rogers is a Research Associate Professor in the Department of Internal Medicine at the University of Michigan.

1

The Reason

I knew a woman who died suddenly of sepsis. That's nothing unusual. In the United States and the world as a whole, sepsis is one of the leading causes of death. But after she died, I took a retrospective look at her life, reconstructing the events that may have contributed to her early death. After she had delivered six children she experienced prolapse of her uterus, and therefore, with medical consultation, she made a decision to have a hysterectomy and oophorectomy. Once her uterus and ovaries were removed she received estrogen replacement therapy, which she took for many years. Estrogen replacement therapy slightly increased her platelet count and after several tests showing elevated platelet counts with an unknown cause, she was given the diagnosis of thrombocytosis. Standard treatment for this disorder at the time was hydroxyurea, which is an antineoplastic drug. Hydroxyurea not only decreases platelet counts, but tends to reduce white blood cell counts, placing her at greater risk of infection. So after years of taking hydroxyurea, she developed an infection at home, which spread to the bloodstream and placed her in the hospital, where she died. Throughout her life, she was a relatively healthy woman—never had cancer or a stroke or a heart attack. But that initial decision she made and each decision along the way were consequential. The hysterectomy and oophorectomy led to estrogen replacement therapy, which led to elevated platelets, which led to a specific diagnosis, which led to hydroxyurea, which led to the infection, which led to death. The points along the way reflect decisions. Was that initial decision a good one? We'll never know. Were there other options along the way that she could have taken? Perhaps. If we had better information from well-conducted studies about the risks and benefits of various therapeutic options and if these options were understandable and accessible at the time, might she be alive today? I think so.

Comparative effectiveness research is a mechanism to provide this needed information. Many people do not know the consequences of various therapies; once diagnosed with a disease, they often rely on professionals for guidance. The ultimate decision is most often made by patients and their families in consultation with physicians and other health care professionals. The choices can be quite daunting—particularly for those patients with scant medical knowledge. Some rely on the advice of a relative or friend who may have had similar experiences. Some turn to media sources such as the Web to search for relevant information.

How would a patient make a good choice? One could imagine that we would gather the relevant facts, lay them all on the table, discuss, debate, and then decide. But where do you obtain these relevant facts? Asking your physician is sensible—but where does each physician obtain this information? The basis of decision making, one would expect, would be driven by empirical evidence: Evidence derived from the results of good quality clinical research studies.

One would hope that there was some grand compendium of knowledge gained from all scientific research that answers every question that each patient has. There isn't. There are guidelines and reviews that compile results from scientific studies for specific conditions. There are trials of various treatments and therapies. There are well-respected medical journals filled with original research articles and reviews related to the detection and treatment of various conditions. But putting all the information together and keeping up-to-date with all the latest studies is a formidable task.

One may be surprised to learn how few studies have been conducted regarding specific therapies and their effects on a person's health. There are too few studies that answer common questions regarding available choices, the timing of such choices, and for whom such choices are relevant. An initial glance at the availability of medical information from media sources might lead one to conclude that we have a wealth of data regarding health and disease. This is true. But most often what one sees are narrative summaries and opinion pieces. Underlying such opinions and narrative reviews, how many original studies have actually been conducted to assess the effects of therapies on specific patient outcomes? Are there studies that indicate whether the therapy works in a wide variety of different types of people, or does it show promise for just certain individuals? It only takes one unexpected diagnosis for you, a family member, or a friend to realize that there are many particular issues regarding disease that we do not yet know. Was there a chance that, somewhere along the line, you could have done something—or avoided something—which could have prevented the diagnosis from occurring? Now that the diagnosis is made, which options are better, knowing that you cannot change your age, your genetic profile, and things that occurred earlier in your life? What is the best decision for me now?

Essentially, **this is a call for actionable intelligence**. We need the type of information that will provide guidance for good decision making for a particular individual at a specific time. This evidence is not regarded as definitive, because additional information can become available over time with each new scientific study. As the results from new studies are published, we have the opportunity to weigh the benefits and harms of alternative methods and to reassess the options.

Comparative effectiveness research provides a refocusing of efforts to answer health questions relevant to individuals in their daily lives. The Institute of Medicine listed this definition of comparative effectiveness research:

> Comparative effectiveness research is the generation and synthesis of evidence that compares the benefits and harms of alternative methods to prevent, diagnose, treat, and monitor a clinical condition or to improve the delivery of care. The purpose of comparative effectiveness research is to assist consumers, clinicians, purchasers, and policy makers to make informed decisions that will improve health care at both the individual and population levels (Institute of Medicine, 2009).

Comparative effectiveness research is intended to assist with health-related decision making that occurs during everyday life. It has been described as answering questions relevant to people in the real world, centering on outcomes that have direct significance to individuals or the population as a whole. Sometimes this type of research is called **patient-centered outcomes research** or patient-centered health research. Because of this, we should be able to provide answers for patients just as they are—with whatever age, gender, background, or medical history they currently have. In essence, this is the "What's best for me?" approach. However, some prefer the term *person-centered*, making the distinction between the patient (only when under medical care) and the person (including all aspects of life in totality, both health and sickness). Frankly, in the real world, such distinctions become a bit blurred in the course of a person's life.

Comparative effectiveness research incorporates study populations that are representative of people seen in clinical practice, focuses on individuals instead of the generalized average patient, and makes a direct comparison between several available treatments or services that are likely to be choices in everyday life. Some call these head-to-head comparisons.

Take A Look

Use your favorite browser to search the Web for a particular disease. Look at ten different sites for this disease. At each of these sites, is the information an opinion piece or a general review? By just reading the information, can you tell where this information comes from? Are there any citations listed? Does the site present an original (new) research study? Become familiar with how to spot original scientific research. Such studies, usually published in scholarly journals, begin with an introduction and a statement of the research question or hypothesis. The methods of the study are explained. This is followed by the results and then a discussion of the findings. Look for original research studies that have been peer-reviewed. Peer review of scholarly research is a process whereby other researchers and experts read the manuscript and evaluate the study prior to publication. The reviewers decide whether the study is of sufficient scientific merit to be published and can suggest changes to improve the methods or reporting of the study. Find five peer-reviewed original research studies.

Comparative effectiveness research has several distinguishing features:

- The intent is to **inform** a specific clinical or health-related decision. These decisions can be at the individual or population levels.
- It involves **comparisons** of viable treatments, services, or policies. These are choices that would be appropriate for individuals or populations—not placebos or sham treatments, as sometimes are used in other types of research. Such comparisons may be of drugs, devices, biologics, procedures such as surgery or radiation, screening tests, behavioral therapies, health policies, and other services or approaches that are intended to improve the health of individuals and populations.
- The focus of the research is within real-world settings or **usual daily life**. The intent is to determine whether health-related choices provide benefit in the context of peoples' lives—not just within a structured research environment. This encompasses information regarding the social environment and involves consideration of behavior and habits. Given the specific condition under investigation, participants in comparative effectiveness studies should reflect the types of people with this condition who are seen during ordinary clinical practice.
- The outcomes are meaningful and **important to patients**. This is a key component. Significant outcomes often relate to how well one functions in life and may include measures such as the ability to perform everyday tasks. These often include measures regarding physical and mental functioning—or deviations from such activities – which would have impact for an individual. Some of these outcomes may be patient reported and therefore, constitute self-reports of symptoms or health-related information. For population studies, outcomes of the policies would have direct relevance and import to the well-being of those affected.
- The research strives to be more **informative at the individual level**. That is, the results of comparative effectiveness research attempt to answer the patient-centered question, "What works best for me?" In the past, research often provided answers for the overall or average patient without enough information to distinguish certain types of patients for whom the therapy might be of particular benefit or harm. For comparative effectiveness research, however, subgroup analyses are encouraged so to better inform specific individuals of likely outcomes. The provision of appropriate information at the individual level may have, collectively, an impact on health measures at the population level as well.

Why?

Put yourself in the shoes of a patient for a moment. Suppose you were planning to see a practitioner for a health-related problem. In an ideal world, what information would you like? Let's make a list of possible questions to elicit answers which may be meaningful and serve as a decision-making aid. Some information may be obtainable from your health care provider and some may require data captured from other sources.

- What are the treatment *options*? I would like to know the entire range of options currently available for this condition.
- What is the *success rate* for these therapies? For each option, what is the likelihood that this treatment will remedy my problem? What percentage of people, when given this therapy, will have resolution of their disorder?
- Are there short-term and/or long-term *benefits* for each option? What beneficial effects can I expect to experience within the next several weeks and over the coming years? Do the short-term or long-term benefits usually occur in almost everyone who chooses this therapy or just in certain people?
- What are the short-term and long-term *adverse* effects for each option? What adverse effects can I expect to experience within the next several weeks and in the years to come? Do the short-term or long-term adverse effects occur rather rarely or commonly in those who choose this option?
- If I start a therapy, how *long* would I likely have to use this therapy? For the next several weeks? For the rest of my life?
- Are there choices regarding *when* this therapy may begin? What are the likely beneficial and/or adverse effects if I start therapy today versus starting six months from now—or a year from now?
- Are there additional tests or procedures to better determine whether I, personally, would *respond* favorably or would likely experience harmful effects for each of the treatment options?
- Where can I go to find additional accurate and reliable *information* regarding these options? Is there information readily available?
- Are there descriptions of other patients' *experiences* for these particular therapies that I could view or is there a way that I can talk with other such patients who have undergone similar experiences?
- As a patient who chooses one of these therapies, what *responsibilities* do I have to ensure the best possible outcomes? Are there different responsibilities based on the option that I choose?
- How much does each of these therapies *cost*? Could I obtain an itemized list with all expected charges? What proportion of these costs will I be required to pay and what proportion will be paid by my medical insurance?
- How long have the practitioners administered these therapies? What is their level of *experience*? What are their success rates?

◘ *Who else* provides these services? Are there several practitioners in my community who deliver similar services? What are their track records?

Feel free to add your own pressing questions to this list. Are there other types of information that you would want before making a decision? Now, step back from the ideal into the real world. How much of this list can you actually obtain in real life? Information regarding the possible range of effects may not be readily available and, sometimes, not all effects—positive or negative—are known. Often, we do not know the exact probability of expected effects. Most clinical trials are short term, so long-term effects may not be fully known. Moreover, questions regarding timing of specific options cannot always be answered with the current published evidence. There are several items on this list that constitute the unknown for a variety of medical conditions.

Decision making can be a complex process. Often data from different sources must be appraised and the manner in which this information is delivered to patients is important. **Health literacy**, or "the degree to which individuals have the capacity to obtain, process, and understand basic health information and services needed to make appropriate health decisions," is critical (Institute of Medicine, 2004). Goals to improve health literacy which are particularly relevant to comparative effectiveness research include (a) developing and disseminating health and safety information that is accurate, accessible, and actionable; (b) promoting changes in the health care delivery system that improve informed decision making; and (c) increasing the dissemination and use of evidence-based health literacy practices and interventions.

There have been considerable efforts to advance communication between patients and health care providers that involve the incorporation of scientific evidence with patient values and preferences. The Informed Medical Decisions Foundation has a number of resources available for patients and practitioners. Decision aids and guides are available. A summary entitled "Shared Decision Making: A Model for Clinical Practice" is available in the *Journal of General Internal Medicine* with practical advice (Elwyn, 2012).

Check It Out
The Centers for Disease Control and Prevention provides an online section regarding health literacy (http://www.cdc.gov/healthliteracy/). Check out their section called "Science Says: Findings You Can Use." Look at some of the approaches that have been useful. Explore how information can be presented (visually, through spoken text, numerical) and tactics for delivering information to enhance understanding.

The objective of comparative effectiveness research is to inform decision making. But the underlying reason, buried beneath these decisions, is the intent to improve peoples' lives. While there are efforts to inform decision making through evidence from the scientific literature, the existing research is not yet deep or wide enough to answer many commonplace questions. In particular, additional comparative effectiveness research studies are needed in the following areas:

- Determination of the long-term effects of therapies and services.
- Tailoring of information to specific attributes of individuals for maximum benefit.
- Mechanisms to inform decision making when the options are complex such as in instances where there are multiple comorbidities, recurrent episodic events with feedback loops, and many diverse time-dependent choices.
- Implementation of therapies in the context of relevant personal values, cultural preferences, and societal norms.
- Development of processes necessary to deliver information in a more timely fashion, especially for new therapies and treatments.

Life involves a series of decisions. While some health-related decisions are straightforward to navigate in the short term, it is difficult to imagine all the eventualities over time. More options present greater challenges. There is some evidence to indicate that people have a difficult time performing three tasks at once, and may have problems when simultaneously attempting decisions that involve three or more elements (Charron and Koechlin, 2010). In addition to inherent physiologic limitations of the brain, even when evidence-based information is available, there may be challenges regarding how this new knowledge is perceived. In fact, the literature regarding cognitive and social influences on decision making is a fascinating area of research in and of itself.

Who Decides?

Historically, the volume and direction of medical research has been a bit lopsided; some areas are researched more than others. At times, this is driven by the interests of the investigators. It also may be the result of the better availability of research funding for particular types of conditions. The prevalence of a problem may influence investigation, with more common disorders yielding a greater concentration of studies. Sometimes the discovery of a novel procedure or product spearheads ancillary applications.

Just as the delivery of medical care tends to be categorized by either type of disease (oncologists for cancer) or body part

Think
Given that every country has limited resources to invest in research, what criteria would you use so that additional medical evidence could be generated? Would you consider the prevalence of a condition or the characteristics of those being treated? Would you consider the degree to which treatments could influence long-term disability? Make a short list of what you would regard as the most important considerations. Also make a list of several factors which would likely place certain types of research at the bottom of your list. That is, which types of research should receive the least attention?

(ophthalmologists for eye disorders or dentists for your teeth), so does the funding of medical research. The National Institutes of Medicine, one of the major funders of medical research, historically has been categorized this way as well. Foundations often follow these same lines—by disease or disorder. Thus, if a researcher wishes to investigate therapies that stretch across body systems or outcomes that affect multiple conditions in individuals, it can be challenging. Since comparative effectiveness research aims to address peoples' choices in the real world, it is important that this point is not lost. People are complex organisms (actually, to be more exact, each person is a mobile ecosystem of organisms interacting with larger networks of ecosystems). Failure to recognize interconnections within the body and larger community influences relevant to both therapies and outcomes may result in missed opportunities in real world settings. Research that addresses complexities is important, and there should be avenues to adequately fund such studies.

Comparative Effectiveness Research in Context

Comparative effectiveness research is broad in scope and multidisciplinary by nature. It can be considered an offshoot of a global movement in evidence-based medicine and interdisciplinary science. Comparative effectiveness research is a subspecialty within both health services research and clinical epidemiology. Some of its roots are in health services research, which brings a set of study designs and decision-making elements relevant to health policy and the delivery of services. Some of its roots are in clinical epidemiology, which serves as a basis for study design, disease measures, and population health science in general. Historically, biostatistics has served a foundational role for both these disciplines and is integrally involved. The methodological underpinnings of comparative effectiveness research are broad so that, at times, studies may include economists, engineers, and computer scientists. Furthermore, because this research involves an examination of real life, methods generated within psychology and sociology often are directly relevant.

Methods for comparative effectiveness research, while often utilized in medicine, have been used by a wide range of health professionals. Dentists, pharmacists, and nurses have employed methods to compare the impacts of therapies or procedures on patient outcomes. In particular, patient functioning and activities of daily living are often selected as patient-centered outcomes in nursing research. Physical therapists, dietitians, speech therapists, and various allied health professionals have used comparative studies to evaluate the effects of services on patient functioning or response to treatment. For example, dietitians have a long history of conducting research of head-to-head comparisons of dietary therapies. Professions typically ancillary to health care may also be involved, particularly since the interventions may have broad applications. If the research involves an educational video or movie, production crews can be team members in the study. If the research involves techniques to abate violence, police and professionals knowledgeable in conflict resolution may be involved.

The conduct of comparative effectiveness research is a team effort. Not every health professional may wish to (or physically could) design a study and implement all aspects of it. There are intentions to more fully develop systems whereby research may be tucked into or integrated within the daily practice of health professionals, with members of the team playing different roles. That is, some health professionals may participate in study design and the development of protocol; others may enroll patients. Clinicians may deliver the therapies while others measure outcomes. The investigative team includes researchers who conduct computerized entry or extraction, and statistical analyses. Even for the retrospective investigations which tap large electronic databases, often multiple professionals are involved with the study design and data analyses. So, while you might not conduct all facets of a study, you may be a critical member of a team that does.

The deliberate effort to use systematic evidence of effectiveness to inform population-based policies and medical decisions has been underway for many years. The Oxford Centre for Evidence-Based Medicine is a major source of information regarding the integration of scientific evidence into clinical practice. The Cochrane Collaboration fulfills an important role worldwide (http://www.cochrane.org/). Researchers at McMaster University in Canada have been on the forefront of evidence-based medicine for decades. There are many centers and governmental agencies throughout the world that have experts in methods central to comparative effectiveness research. Among them are the US Preventive Services Task Force, the Canadian Agency for Drugs and Technologies in Health Care, the National Institute for Health and Clinical Excellence (NICE) in the United Kingdom, and the Institute for Quality and Efficiency in Health Care in Germany. The volume of agencies intrinsically involved with the integration of medical evidence into clinical practices has expanded worldwide and is constantly evolving. International organizations have been formed, such as the International Network of Agencies for Health Technology Assessment, which have a common mission to share information regarding the effectiveness of various medical interventions.

At first glance, one might think that this type of research is best left to far-off experts who live and practice somewhere else. Not so. This type of integrative research can be generated by various health professionals in the course of everyday practice. The objectives are broad, as are the methods and applications. There are opportunities for participation by clinicians and, most critically, for all of us patients. We are in the center of this. Don't sit back and just hope that your health questions will be answered by someone else. We are all a part of this. If we want answers to our questions, we have to step up to the plate.

2

The Question

> "I have a friend in college who had juvenile diabetes since he was five years old. So I am interested in studying type 1 diabetes."
>
> "What do you want to know about it?"
>
> "Well, it was kind of tough for him. He had all these great resources for managing his diabetes when he was a kid but when he was out on his own, things changed. After leaving home, he had a hard time finding someone who really knows a lot about insulin dosing in young adults and his—you know—day-to-day issues. Just getting all his supplies was a problem. Isn't there a better way of changing over from pediatrics to adult care?"
>
> "I certainly don't know the answer to that one. Did you ask around?"
>
> "Yeah, but I couldn't find much. Not the kind of information that I wanted."

Research studies often start with interest and a problem worth solving. This interest is then translated into a framework, which outlines the aspects of the issues that are germane to the problem. This can form the nucleus for a formal investigation.

A scientific study starts with a specific aim, hypothesis, or research question. This directs the study and determines elements of its design. In the conversion above, it is clear who constitutes the population of interest: young adults with type 1 diabetes mellitus. The question, as posed, indicates an interest in "methods of transition," which would be various approaches relating to the continuity of care (from pediatrics to adult care). Various methods of transition could potentially form the interventions or comparators, because the researcher would be examining different approaches to managing transition. Possible patient-centered outcomes would then be explored. What are the important aspects of life which may be improved by smoothing this transition?

The ability to translate an issue or problem into a meaningful question has considerable import for the conduct of research. The formulation of a clinical question for research purposes has been enhanced by the acronym PICO, which stands for Population, Intervention, Comparison, and Outcome:

- **Population.** Who are the individuals to be studied? Should they represent particular types of people (by age, gender, condition, or other factors)? To whom would I want to refer the study results?
- **Intervention.** What therapy, procedure, service, preventive measure, or other intervention do I wish to study?
- **Comparison.** What are the comparison groups? Will this be a head-to-head comparison of two different treatments or does this comparison involve three or four approaches? In comparative effectiveness research, there may be instances in which both the intervention and all the comparators are of equal interest (all may be labeled comparators without using the term intervention or intervention group). In other instances, there may be a notable difference between the new treatment (labeled the intervention) and the comparison treatment (labeled the comparator).
- **Outcome.** What is the primary outcome for this study? What are the other outcomes? In comparative effectiveness research, often outcomes that are patient reported are included and the investigators may choose to report the entire range of outcomes that pertain to each of the treatments under study.

Sometimes the acronym PICOTS is used, whereby the PICO is represented by the items above, and "T" stands for timing and "S" for setting. Timing allows the investigators to specify design elements related to the timing of the intervention and comparators, as well as the timing of the outcome measures. Setting allows specification of the investigation to specific locations and/or practices relevant to either the providers or the participants.

By defining these elements, the intent of the study should be clear. Studies that use each of these elements within the research question provide clarity to the investigators developing the study, to participants within the study, and to the intended audiences after the study is completed. It is important to specify who will be studied, the comparisons being made, and the outcomes measured.

In the chapters to come, comparators and outcomes will be examined in more detail. We will also explore more details regarding the population or patients, the setting or place, and timing. In epidemiology, the infusion of person, place, and time into research has been a cornerstone of practice. When formulating a research question in comparative effectiveness research, these elements are important.

Try This
Go online to the TRIP database (http://www.tripdatabase.com/). On the main page, you'll see an option called "PICO search." Type in whatever options you wish in the four search boxes and see what types of articles are retrieved. This is another way to search the biomedical literature for a given research question.

> **Consider**
> Below are examples of aims and research questions that lack clarity. Which PICO items are missing? What items would be necessary for comparative effectiveness research?
> - We intend to study how families with autistic children cope.
> - Does increasing daily protein intake reduce weight gain?
> - Does walking reduce the risk of Alzheimer's disease?

In effect, a well-defined research question constitutes an expression of study intent. When a project is being proposed or submitted for funding purposes, some researchers may have an option to restate the research question into a specific aim or specific hypotheses. **A scientific hypothesis is a working assumption that is tested in a study.** Often in comparative effectiveness research, the hypothesis is an assumption of the likely relative effectiveness of one therapy versus another. The elements included in the hypothesis are specific enough such that, at the end of the study, one can conduct a test to evaluate the probability that this hypothesis is likely to be true.

An example of a specific aim may be:

- We will compare the degree to which the Grenndon Therapy and Hilswarch Approach affect the severity of postpartum fatigue, as measured by the Visual Analogue of Fatigue Scale in multiparous women 16–45 years of age, in the 30 days after delivery.

For this same study, the research question would be:

- Does the Grenndon Therapy have a different effect on the severity of postpartum fatigue than the Hilswarch Approach in the 30 days after delivery, as measured by the Visual Analogue of Fatigue Scale in multiparous women 16–45 years of age?

The hypothesis for this same study is most often stated as a null hypothesis for direct assessment in a statistical test. That is, the null hypothesis would be:

- There is no difference in mean severity of postpartum fatigue between the Grenndon Therapy and the Hilswarch Approach in the 30 days after delivery, as measured by the Visual Analogue of Fatigue Scale in multiparous women 16–45 years of age.

Many scientists are accustomed to formally testing hypotheses, so the null hypothesis should look familiar. If you are not yet accustomed to this approach, it is quite understandable in a general sense. Take the "no difference in mean severity of postpartum fatigue" that was stated above. We would measure the mean severity of fatigue in the women receiving the Grenndon Therapy. Then we would measure the mean severity of fatigue in women receiving the Hilswarch Approach. Subtract the two means to find the difference. We can ascertain how likely this difference is by comparing it to known distributions of what differences generally look like in populations. This gives us a sense of how rare our findings are. If the mean difference in severity were small, we would be more likely to say that there is no difference in the effect of the Grenndon Therapy versus the Hilswarch Approach (and we would not reject the null hypothesis). If the mean difference were large, we would be more likely to say—wow! It does make a difference.

Standards for Formulating Research Questions

The **Patient-Centered Outcomes Research Institute** (PCORI) facilitates evidence-based research to assist individuals with making health care decisions. Their standards for formulating research questions are as follows:

- Identify gaps in evidence.
- Develop a formal study protocol.
- Identify specific populations and health decisions affected by the research.
- Identify and assess participant subgroups.
- Select appropriate interventions and comparators.
- Measure outcomes that people representing the population of interest notice and care about.

> **Take A Look**
>
> Go to the Patient-Centered Outcomes Research Institute (PCORI) site (http://www.pcori.org/). Look at the types of research being funded. What research questions did these studies ask? Explore the site. Also visit the "Get Involved" section. There is an option called Suggest Topics where you can suggest a patient-centered research question. On this page, the instructions indicate, "Whether you are a patient with a health condition, a caregiver for someone else, a health care professional who wants to improve care for your patients, or a researcher, we invite you to submit a question. In addition to questions about options faced by patients, we also are interested in questions that would help to improve health care delivery, address disparities in health care, or improve the communication of research findings." Within the next 3 months as you explore comparative effectiveness research in more detail, think about possible questions that may be of interest to you. If you have a good idea or a particular question of interest, go ahead and submit it directly on this PCORI site (http://www.pcori.org/get-involved/suggest-a-patient-centered-research-question-survey/).

Research questions are often influenced by priorities set through funding agencies, institutes, or federal sources. In some countries, national priorities for health-related research are generated. In the United States, a list of priority topics was developed and they are organized by quartile ranking (Institute of Medicine, 2009). For example, one of the initial national priorities for comparative effectiveness research in the United States is listed below:

> Compare the effectiveness of various primary care treatment strategies (e.g., symptom management, cognitive behavior therapy, biofeedback, social skills, educator/teacher training, parent training, pharmacologic treatment) for attention deficit hyperactivity disorder (ADHD) in children.

> **Practice**
> Try translating these two priorities into PICOTS-type questions. You will need to select strategies and explore outcomes relevant to the conditions under investigation. Consider the types of information required to build such questions.

Here is another initial national priority:

Compare the effectiveness of different strategies of introducing biologics into the treatment algorithm for inflammatory diseases, including Crohn's disease, ulcerative colitis, rheumatoid arthritis, and psoriatic arthritis.

Searching the Literature

One of the first steps in exploring an issue and developing a framework is to investigate the research that has already been conducted in that particular area. Researchers should know how to perform a thorough search of the biomedical literature to retrieve information regarding previous studies that have been published relevant to their hypotheses.

A bibliographic database is a repository that contains references to journal articles and other published literature. In comparative effectiveness research, it is important to review previous biomedical research that is published in scientific journals. Often the citation and the abstract are housed within the repository. There are several large bibliographic databases that are frequently used by health researchers:

- MEDLINE is a bibliographic database that was created by the US National Library of Medicine. It houses journal citations and abstracts of journal articles that were published in the life sciences with a particular concentration in biomedicine. Indexing of the records is through a hierarchical system of Medical Subject Headings (MeSH).
- Embase is a repository of scientific studies containing entries related to biomedical research including pharmacologic studies. It is particularly important for researchers interested in drug therapies. Although it is not open-access, it may be available through certain libraries.
- The Cochrane Library is a compendium of six different databases and includes the Cochrane database of systematic reviews, the Cochrane central register of controlled trials, the Cochrane methodology register, the database of abstracts of reviews of effects, the health technology assessment database, and the National Health System economic evaluation database. The Cochrane Library is available through paid subscription in some countries and regions while in others, it is openly available to users online (search for access options for the Cochrane Library to see the countries with open access).
- The Cumulative Index to Nursing and Allied Health Literature (CINAHL) is available generally through libraries, for those

researchers interested in interventions related to nursing practice and the allied health professions. Searching is through subject headings similar to that used by the US National Library of Medicine.
- PsycINFO is a database of citations and abstracts of the peer-reviewed literature (journals, books, dissertations) and contains studies regarding psychology, behavioral sciences, and mental health. It is available through subscription and is often accessible through academic libraries.
- The Education Resources Information Center (ERIC) is useful for finding educational resources relevant to health, and may be particularly important if you are working with therapies that involve an educational component. It is a freely accessible online database of published educational literature including journal articles, conference papers, and dissertations (http://www.eric.ed.gov/). Some full-text articles are also available.
- The Physiotherapy Evidence Database (http://www.pedro.org.au) contains citations and abstracts of trials, systematic reviews, and practice guidelines related to physiotherapy. Online searching is freely available.
- Scopus, Biological Abstracts, and Web of Science are general databases of the scientific literature. They are available by subscription and are often accessible through academic libraries.
- If you are interested in nutrition and dietary interventions, you might try the freely available AGRIS, the International Information System for the Agricultural Sciences and Technology by the Food and Agriculture Organization of the United Nations (http://agris.fao.org/), or AGRICOLA at the US Department of Agriculture (http://agricola.nal.usda.gov/). Both offer free searches online.
- There are studies which utilize information technology applications in health care and for these researchers, the open-access Collection of Computer Science Bibliographies may be helpful (http://liinwww.ira.uka.de/bibliography/). If you select the Browse option, the subject areas are listed.
- There are general collections of digital library resources available at the WorldCat database (http://www.worldcat.org/). It is a catalog of digital resources and includes citations for journal articles, books, and other published literature, as well as DVDs and CDs. Searching is freely available online.
- For researchers interested in economic aspects of health care, RePEc, Research Papers in Economics (http://repec.org/), houses an open-access bibliographic database. Journal articles, working papers, software, and books can be freely searched.
- If you are working in injury research, SafetyLit is a bibliographic database with a search engine and is freely available online (http://

www.safetylit.org/). It includes journal articles, reports, and doctoral theses regarding risk factors for injury, the epidemiology of injury, and societal consequences of injury.
- A bibliographic database called Scientific Electronic Library Online (SciELO) contains journal articles, including biomedical publications, from many developing countries and its services are freely available online (http://www.scielo.org/php/index.php?lang=en).
- The Social Science Research Network houses a large searchable open-access bibliographic repository for those health researchers interested in social aspects of health and disease (http://www.ssrn.com/). It contains some helpful features such as readily available suggested citation, email addresses of authors, and easily downloadable papers in pdf format when available.

Beyond the bibliographic databases, there are systems and search engines that allow access to databases and facilitate searching. PubMed was developed at the US National Library of Medicine and allows for free access to MEDLINE and full-text articles in PubMed Central (http://www.ncbi.nlm.nih.gov/pubmed). Commercial searching products are available as well through subscription, such as Ovid which offers access to MEDLINE, PsycINFO, Embase, and other repositories. In addition, there are online search engines available to locate biomedical original research articles. The Directory of Open Access Journals is a useful site (http://www.doaj.org/) because you can pull up the full-text articles for research studies published in open-access journals. Scirus provides access to a large volume of scientific literature (>575 million entries) and allows free searching by abstracts, articles, dissertations, books, conferences, patents, and other published literature (http://www.scirus.com/). My search for care transitions AND "type 1 diabetes" yielded 5925 hits, with meaningful entries listed. Another option is CiteSeer^x, which is an open-access academic search engine for finding citations in information science (allowing metadata harvesting) and may be useful for information technology applications in health care (http://citeseerx.ist.psu.edu/index). It is a slightly different application in that it incorporates algorithms and techniques useful in extracting and manipulating data from digital repositories. BASE (Bielefeld Academic Search Engine) is an open-access search engine for academic research and will allow searching by article, theses, and other digital documents including images, audio, video, and software (http://www.base-search.net/). Google Scholar is an open-access search engine of journal articles, reports, theses, and other scientific literature and provides citation indexing so that abstracts of cited articles can be readily accessed. Microsoft Academic Search is another search engine for journal articles with a time-relevant visualization tool for publications and citations. For those interested in genetic studies, Bioinformatic Harvester (http://harvester.

Try This

In the opening scenario, there was an interest in care transitions for young adults with type 1 diabetes mellitus. Let's use this example to search for original research on this topic.

- Search for PubMed online (http://www.ncbi.nlm.nih.gov/pubmed). Go to the site and you will see "Clinical Queries" which is listed under PubMed Tools on the main page. Select this. In the search box within PubMed Clinical Queries, type in "care transitions" and then examine the studies which are displayed at the bottom of the page. The results are categorized into clinical studies, systematic reviews, and medical genetics. If you select filter information at the bottom of each category, the search strategies for obtaining these articles are listed. Note that, for the clinical studies, you can select articles that deal with therapy, diagnosis, etiology, prognosis, or clinical prediction guides. Now, try narrowing our search to care transitions AND "type 1 diabetes." Do you find any information regarding transitioning of care in type 1 diabetes?

- Go to PubMed Central (http://www.ncbi.nlm.nih.gov/pmc/). Try typing the phrase we used earlier: care transitions AND "type 1 diabetes." Note the number of hits from this search. When you select one of the studies, notice that the entire article is available. There are several ways to view the article including a PubReader and as a pdf file. You could also try using HubMed, which is labeled "PubMed rewired" and allows you to search in a slightly different manner. Go to HubMed (http://www.hubmed.org) and type in care transitions AND "type 1 diabetes." If you select some of the articles, you can display a TouchGraph of the articles.

- Next, go to Europe PubMed Central (http://europepmc.org/) and search for the same phrase: care transitions AND "type 1 diabetes." How many articles were retrieved at this site? On the right-hand side, you can select meta-analyses, randomized clinical trials, or all clinical trials. Scan some of these publications and start to gain some perspective on what aspects of care transition are known in type 1 diabetes.

- Next try the Cochrane Library, which is a collection of biomedical databases of health-related studies. Search for it online (http://www.thecochranelibrary.com/view/0/index.html). Type in the same phrase regarding care transitions AND "type 1 diabetes." What do you find?

- Now try the TRIP database (http://www.tripdatabase.com/). When you go to this site, the search box is right in front of you so you can type in the same diabetes phrase as above. What do you find? Note that you can further refine your results by type (secondary evidence which includes reviews and guidelines, key primary research or controlled trials, etc.). In addition, there are other mechanisms to categorize the results by the options listed across the top running bar (evidence, images, videos, education, patient information, news, PubMed Clinical Queries, DynaMed). DynaMed is a tool for providing evidence-based summaries for clinicians to facilitate decision making.

- Another readily available source of information is the searchable Education Resources Information Center (http://www.eric.ed.gov). Try typing in "care transitions" in the search box. Take a look at the types of articles it retrieves. If you cannot find many innovative ideas regarding transitional care in the usual medical databases, try looking at something like this, in which transitions have been studied in greater depth but in different contexts. You probably will not find many specific applications listed for type 1 diabetes *per se*. But it can spark ideas regarding applications that you may wish to explore in a clinical investigation.

- You might also try searching for the same diabetes phrase using BASE (http://www.base-search.net/), which is an open-access academic search engine originating from the Bielefeld University Library. Search for "BASE search engine." Then type in care transitions AND "type 1 diabetes" and compare the results retrieved during this search.

kit.edu/HarvesterPortal) is freely available for searching genes and proteins, as well as relevant scientific publications.

Searching the biomedical literature is not only a good start in terms of reviewing previous findings, but it can also give you an idea of how researchers frame a question and how they conduct particular types of studies. Exposure to many research studies—especially good-quality studies—can be enlightening. Reading original research studies can provide insights into the types of questions that can be answered and the methods available for investigation.

When you go to PubMed and select an article, you might notice that, in some instances, you will be able to see the entire article. For studies that were funded by the US National Institutes of Health, open access to the public becomes available after a certain period of time in subscription journals. To directly see the entire article for a given search on a topic, try PubMed Central (http://www.ncbi.nlm.nih.gov/pmc/). PubMed Central is different than PubMed. PubMed Central is a free archive of the medical literature and contains the full text of each publication.

In addition, the National Institute for Health and Care Excellence (NICE) in the United Kingdom has an easy-to-search site that allows for filtering by clinical queries, types of information, or sources (https://www.evidence.nhs.uk/). An evidence search for care transitions in type 1 diabetes at this site yielded many specific articles on this topic.

If you are interested in radiology or one of the basic sciences and will be assessing technologies for their health applications, you might try the Science Accelerator, which is an open-access search engine to scientific research hosted by the Department of Energy (http://www.scienceaccelerator.gov/). These sources represent a broader variety of articles, but when you are in an exploratory phase and have not quite decided on all aspects of your investigation, this could generate some ideas. Another yet broader scientific database is the global search engine that can be found at WorldWideScience (http://www.worldwidescience.org). This site allows for multilingual translation searching.

After investigating the digital repositories, think about aspects in which these sites are similar and also reflect on elements that are distinctive and particularly useful. Perhaps you could suggest some improvements that would relate to how the search terms are entered or how the results are displayed. If you were to design the perfect strategy for extracting and utilizing findings from previous biomedical research, how would this strategy be different from the systems available today?

3

The Choice

Each day we make choices affecting our health—from the choice to use an alarm clock to force us out of bed, to the foods we choose to eat or avoid at breakfast, and to the way we use the elevator to circumvent the stairway on the way to our seventh-floor office. There are a multitude of instinctive choices that we make throughout the course of a day.

These are the usual choices. Now think about things that do not occur during a typical day for most people, such as an occasional injury or illness. I wrenched my shoulder and it hurts. Take a pain pill? Sit down for a while and hope that it stops? Call my doctor? Stop by urgent care? Don't worry about it—just suffer through and get back to work? Making wise choices is important. While some decisions may not have great long-term impact, other health decisions can have grave consequences. Being able to have the information necessary to make wise choices is an integral part of comparative effectiveness research.

Try This
Make a list of ten choices that you make during a typical day that probably affect your mental or physical well-being, directly or indirectly.

Incorporating evidence into everyday practices is an ongoing challenge. One such effort was advanced by the National Physicians Alliance, and is called Choosing Wisely˚. Patients and physicians are being encouraged to have conversations regarding health choices (www.choosingwisely.org). To start the conversation, specific issues are being addressed in the light of current scientific evidence. These issues relate to the necessity of some medical practices, and were meant to initiate discussions regarding whether or not certain procedures would be a wise choice. For example, a few items on the list are:

- Don't order antibiotics for adenoviral conjunctivitis (pink eye).
- Don't do imaging for uncomplicated headache.
- Cough and cold medicines should not be prescribed or recommended for respiratory illnesses in children under four years of age.
- Avoid cardiovascular testing for patients undergoing low-risk surgery.
- Avoid nonsteroidal anti-inflammatory drugs (NSAIDs) in individuals with hypertension or heart failure or chronic kidney disease of all causes, including diabetes.

- Don't schedule elective, non-medically indicated inductions of labor or Cesarean deliveries before 39 weeks, 0 days gestational age.
- Don't obtain imaging studies in patients with non-specific low back pain.
- Don't prescribe testosterone to men with erectile dysfunction who have normal testosterone levels.
- Don't recommend percutaneous feeding tubes in patients with advanced dementia; instead offer oral assisted feeding.
- Don't screen for carotid artery stenosis (CAS) in asymptomatic adult patients.
- Don't perform Pap smears on women younger than 21 or who have had a hysterectomy for non-cancer disease.
- Don't routinely use bronchodilators in children with bronchiolitis.
- Don't use PET/CT for cancer screening in healthy individuals.

Explore
Go online and read through other Choosing Wisely® recommendations. Also look at the short descriptions after each recommendation, which give the reasons why these choices were advised. Were you aware of any of these recommendations? Are some of these surprising to you?

The key to such recommendations is an evaluation of the research evidence for and against certain therapies and an assessment based on the totality of evidence. This information originates from research studies, which compare various treatment choices and report patient outcomes associated with these therapies. Let's explore the various categories of choices that one could evaluate to see if they work to relieve symptoms, improve functioning, or affect well-being. We begin with a few common terms which are important to understand in this research framework.

Efficacy and Effectiveness

Within the context of clinical research, efficacy and effectiveness have specific definitions. Efficacy refers to whether an intervention produces an effect under ideal or controlled conditions. Effectiveness refers to whether an intervention produces an effect in ordinary life or in routine clinical practice. Efficacy answers the question, "Can it work?" while effectiveness answers the question, "Does it work in routine care?" Efficacy of an intervention usually is tested using a double-blind randomized controlled trial. Effectiveness of an intervention can be assessed in various trials or comparison studies in which the treatments and effects more closely match real-world occurrences. A double-blind randomized controlled trial of a new antihistamine versus placebo would assess efficacy. A nonrandomized open-label trial of a new antihistamine compared to a steroid nasal spray in adult patients with allergies would assess effectiveness.

One of the ways in which efficacy and effectiveness studies differ is in the participants who are selected for the study. Often in efficacy trials, the inclusion criteria are more stringent. Allowing patients with more complex conditions into the trial may create difficulties in the interpretation of the results. Patients with multiple and diverse preexisting conditions may have different or unanticipated reactions to the drugs under study, and the response to the investigative drug may be muted or enhanced compared to patients who have fewer comorbidities. These differing effects have implications for the analyses, interpretation of the results, and conclusions. For efficacy studies, often the choice is made to use a more homogenous group of participants in which to formally test a therapy. An effectiveness study, on the other hand, is generally more inclusive. The participants in the study are more similar to the types of patients in whom this therapy is likely to benefit and for whom it may be utilized during routine clinical practice.

Another way in which efficacy trials sometimes differ from effectiveness studies is the comparison group. In efficacy trials, a placebo can be used as the comparator. In drug trials, this enables the researcher to incorporate blinding of the participants and the investigators to which drug (active treatment or placebo) is being used in the various groups. However, in ordinary life, most patients are faced with a comparison between alternative therapies. For example, they could immediately start drug therapy or they could begin a weight loss management program. Which is better? An effectiveness trial could pit initiation of drug therapy against the weight loss program.

Efficacy trials, as opposed to effectiveness studies, generally employ more robust study design. Under ideal conditions, will this therapy work? Care is taken to keep all extraneous factors as similar as possible—except for the receipt of the intervention. This enables a more clear comparison and a straightforward statistical analysis. Effectiveness studies, however, can be conducted using several different designs. Sometimes they are trials. Randomization may or may not be employed. Sometimes they are prospective cohort studies, observing individuals who received several different treatments over a particular period of time. There is a basic comparison, but if randomization is not utilized, extra effort must be made to deal with potential extraneous factors that may influence the interpretation of the results and conclusions.

Issues with Placebos as Comparators

A placebo is a drug without active ingredients, or a nontherapeutic procedure or strategy that is not perceived to provide medical benefit. Placebos are used in medical research to provide an assessment of patient outcomes without the drug or procedure of interest. They are used to evaluate the background rates of patient outcomes compared to the rates of outcomes when an active ingredient of a medication is used or when a sham or nontherapeutic procedure is performed.

Why not use a placebo in comparative effectiveness research? Since the goal of comparative effectiveness research is to provide information regarding choices in medical care that are applicable to the daily lives of individuals, placebos are not a typical treatment choice. Head-to-head comparisons of the types of treatments likely to provide benefit may provide meaningful information regarding effects experienced in the context of usual care. This, in essence, is the rationale for comparative effectiveness research.

Issues with Usual Care as a Comparator

In some research studies, the comparison group is defined as usual care. So why not compare a new treatment to usual care? The answer to this is straightforward: because "usual care" is often not a single entity and may be difficult to define. It can vary from one practitioner to the next, or from hospital to hospital. Variation in medical practices has been extensively documented. The *Dartmouth Atlas of Health Care* chronicles this in the United States (http://www.dartmouthatlas.org/). Hospital use, surgical procedures, and care of individuals with chronic illness vary significantly across regions. International differences have also been documented.

If a study were to be conducted in which unspecified usual care were compared with a treatment, conclusions and recommendations at the end of the study may be difficult to explain. What were the elements that constituted usual care in this study? Were they uniformly administered? However, if the investigators meticulously defined the elements of such usual care and incorporated these elements uniformly, then the definition of their comparator becomes informative. By providing details regarding this comparator, it can become a viable alternative.

It is also possible that the alternative is labeled as "watchful waiting" or "watch and wait." In this instance, a treatment is not given at a specific time and monitoring of a patient's status may involve repeated testing over time with the stipulation that, if changes occur in the patient's status, treatment would commence at that time. If this comparator is chosen, the parameters of watchful waiting should be defined. This would include information regarding the time period utilized, the level of monitoring, and the specific criteria in which the waiting would be stopped to allow for the initiation of treatment. Therefore, similar to the choice of usual care, the choice of watchful waiting only becomes meaningful in comparative effectiveness research when the exact specifications are delineated and they are uniformly applied when the research study is conducted. Watchful waiting can be a viable comparator when appropriately defined.

The following paragraphs describe the types of comparators that are often utilized within comparative effectiveness research. Since the methods of comparative effectiveness research are broad, it is useful to examine the range of comparators available for this type of research. Note that the word "comparators" refers to all the viable options being considered or tested in a study.

Medications as Comparators

One of the most common treatments for disease is medication. What are the expected benefits and risks of a specific drug? If there are several medications on the market for a particular condition, which medication would be most beneficial for me? When is it appropriate to begin taking the drug? When it is beneficial to increase or decrease the dosage? Are there other nonmedication therapies that may have desirable effects and would be viable alternatives? How will this drug interact with the other medications that I take? What are the adverse effects of the medication, and how does this impact my decision to continue on this medication or to use another? There are numerous questions that patients ask regarding medications. While there may be evidence-based information to answer some of these questions, in almost all instances, we would benefit from additional information regarding benefits, risks, timing, and alternatives.

In most countries, there is a governmental body that provides oversight regarding the safety of medications. In the United States, the Food and Drug Administration is responsible for oversight regarding drug safety, while in the United Kingdom, it is the Medicines and Healthcare Products Regulatory Agency. Australia has its Therapeutic Goods Administration, while in Canada, drug regulations fall under the jurisdiction of Health Canada. Other countries have similar agencies at the national level for monitoring and regulating prescription medications. In addition, international umbrella organizations have been developed, such as the European Medicines Agency for drug regulation within the European Union. Information from federal agencies can serve as an instructional guide, since often both provider and consumer information is available.

In general, human clinical trials of drugs follow a natural progression, starting with smaller studies designed to evaluate safety and continuing with larger studies that assess both safety and efficacy. The evaluation of new drugs generally follows a pathway of phased trials, and these phases are listed online at the clinical trial website (http://clinicaltrials.gov/ct2/help/glossary/phase) in the United States. Such trials begin with exploratory investigational new drug studies (Phase 0) and progress to small studies of drug adverse effects and mechanisms related to absorption, metabolism, and excretion (Phase 1); small trials of the efficacy and safety of drugs using a control group (Phase 2); large randomized controlled trials of the efficacy and safety of drugs (Phase 3); and studies that assess safety,

> **Discover**
>
> Use your favorite search engine to learn more about the phases of clinical trials. Which of the phases are most similar to (or overlap with) comparative effectiveness research? The Cochrane Central Register for Controlled Trials (CENTRAL), International Clinical Trials Registry Platform of the World Health Organization, the Clinicaltrials.gov, and CenterWatch.com are central sites for registering clinical trials. Look at a few of the existing clinical trials online at these sites. Can you list a few studies that may qualify as comparative effectiveness research in terms of having two or more nonplacebo comparators, and which assess outcomes that directly relate to possible benefits to people in their daily lives?

effects, cost, and utilization of drugs after they are approved and available for use to the wider public (Phase 4). This last phase is sometimes called postmarketing surveillance.

Many medication trials are conducted by pharmaceutical companies when bringing new drugs to the market. However, there are instances in which not all possible comparisons have been assessed in these trials including studies using non-drug related comparators. Moreover, not all trials include patients who may be similar to those who might possibly benefit from this treatment. Older adults and children tend to be disproportionately excluded from randomized controlled trials (Van Spall, 2007). Historically there were fewer women in clinical trials than men, with some concerns regarding possible safety issues for women of childbearing age. There also have been fewer clinical trials with individuals who have multiple diseases or who have complex clinical profiles, because concomitant use of differing medications may be problematic when assessing single drug effects. However, one could make the case that it is precisely in these types of patients in which both providers and patients need more information regarding effectiveness. It is important to determine which combinations of medications work well in patients with complex conditions and to clarify the range of different types of people (both young and old) who are likely in need of such therapies. Gaps in knowledge regarding drug use involve insufficient information regarding:

> **Explore**
>
> The Food and Drug Administration provides an Online Label Repository (http://labels.fda.gov/). Go to this site and click on Proprietary Name Search. Type in any drug name that you wish. Read the recommendations and contraindications listed for this drug. Were you aware that this detailed information was readily available? You might also try the Active Ingredient Search to discover different drugs with similar active ingredients. In addition, by selecting the Drugs tab at the top crossbar, you can explore the types of information available on drugs for health professionals and consumers. Information is given regarding safety, availability, approvals and databases, compliance and regulations, emergency preparedness, and research.

- head-to-head comparisons with other drugs currently on the market or other non-drug treatment approaches;
- adverse and beneficial effects in certain types of patients (e.g., children, women, people with multiple conditions, people of different genetic profiles or family histories);
- long-term use;
- timing of administration.

Often both beneficial and harmful effects are studied in the context of Phase 3 randomized controlled trials. However, there are instances in which a medication is found to be safe and efficacious from a double-blind randomized controlled trial and after the drug is marketed to the larger population, other effects of the drug become evident. *Adverse effects* are those in which the patient is harmed in some way. *Side effects* of a drug are those that are secondary to the main intent of the drug. Side effects can be either beneficial or harmful to the patient.

Medical Devices as Comparators

Medical devices constitute a wide range of products—generally instruments, tools, and machines that are utilized for health-related purposes. There is a considerable array of devices that have health-related applications, but they are often distinguished from medications in that drugs act through chemical means, whereby devices act through physical means. Think back to your basic sciences. Chemistry yields the medications, physics yields the devices, and biology yields the biologics—any of which may serve as a comparator in research. Moreover, through technology there can be combinations of therapies that reach across disciplines. The drug-eluting vascular stent is an example of a physical device with a chemical component.

Devices are widely utilized in health care settings and in the home. Some are quite simple, such as a bandage. Others are complex, such as the membrane lung for long-term pulmonary support in neonates, which provides extracorporeal membrane oxygenation. Some are external to the patient's body and are utilized to gather data regarding metrics relevant to underlying physiologic processes, such as the commonly used sphygmomanometer and blood pressure cuff. Others may be implanted internally, such as a hip joint prosthesis used in total hip arthroplasty. Some devices are designed to be used for insertion in and out of the body, such as the intermittent urinary catheter. There are devices that operate using radio frequency telemetry such as a wireless pacemaker or a wireless insulin pump. Some emit ionizing radiation such as X-rays, or utilize sound waves such as ultrasound. Some devices are expansive and are housed at specific sites—such as the magnetic resonance imaging (MRI) scanner—while others are small and available over-the-counter, like a thermometer sold at the corner drug store.

Medical devices are often categorized into various classes by regulatory agencies. Class I devices are the least risky (think tongue depressors), and as class levels increase, so does risk. Examples of

Discover
The Food and Drug Administration oversees medical device safety in the United States. Go to their site and locate the medical device section. Search for "device classification panels" (http://www.fda.gov/MedicalDevices/ DeviceRegulationandGuidance/Overview/ ClassifyYourDevice/ucm051530.htm). The Device Classification Panels page provides a list of devices categorized by medical specialty. Click on some of the choices given by each medical specialty. Look at the types of devices listed. See if you can find ten devices which you never heard of before.

Class I medical devices include an irrigating syringe, a suction snakebite kit, a neonatal eyepad, and a manual colony counter in microbiology. Examples of typical Class II devices are a low-level laser system for aesthetic use, a bone sonometer, an electrocardiograph, and a porcelain tooth. Examples of Class III devices are an indwelling blood oxyhemoglobin concentration analyzer, a ventricular bypass assist device, a testicular prosthesis, and an implanted intracerebral/subcortical stimulator for pain relief.

Often, the company that manufactures the device will conduct studies regarding the accuracy of the device, as well as studies regarding satisfaction and feasibility of use for health care professionals and patients. However, for many medical devices, there is no governmental requirement to conduct human studies to demonstrate safety or effectiveness. Clinical studies of safety or efficacy may be required for some Class II devices, but not all. In the United States, it is required that Class III devices undergo clinical studies to demonstrate safety and efficacy.

Comparative effectiveness research can perform an important role in the evaluation of devices. For many medical devices, information may not be available regarding the patient-level effects compared to other options. Sometimes this is not considered of grave concern, because the device is so commonly used and appears to serve its designated function. But even the most common device—such as examination gloves—can present an opportunity for study. Do vinyl or latex gloves allow more leakage of viruses? Do the rates of allergic reactions in glove wearers vary between vinyl and latex?

For some studies of medical devices, it may be an evaluation of what the device delivers rather than the device itself. One standard therapy available in medicine involves radiation. Comparative effectiveness studies which contrast various types of radiation therapies regarding the frequency of timing or dosages are possible, as are studies comparing radiation to other approaches such as specific chemotherapeutic agents.

Each year, there are many new medical devices that are available to consumers. The volume of such new devices and the fact that not all medical devices are required to undergo randomized controlled trial testing in humans provides an opportunity for comparative effectiveness research. A useful starting place for such research is to examine medical device registries. Increasingly, more devices are being given a unique identification number, and when a patient receives the device with this identification number, he or she is registered with other such patients and information is collected over time regarding patient-relevant effects and/or device-related malfunctions. Large electronic registries of such patients with similar devices can constitute an important avenue for investigation because the event rates for adverse effects can be readily generated. If the rate of adverse events is elevated for a particular device or if an unexpected beneficial side effect occurs in a particular group of patients, these findings may spur further investigation and action. If the outcomes demonstrate variability across certain recipient characteristics, this too could serve as a starting point for further study; which recipients received the greatest benefit? The use of device registries can provide an important mechanism for advancing knowledge in this field. Some have advocated that such registries should not be too specific. Narrow registries may be less useful in the discovery of common effects across devices with similar attributes. For example, finding that the leaching of a specific metal in a particular device might spur an investigator to look at other devices containing this particular metal.

Discover
Some countries and international entities have developed registries for medical devices. For example, the Therapeutic Goods Administration of the Australian Government has set up a reporting mechanism for medical devices (http://www.tga.gov.au/safety/problem.htm). Check out how it captures information for patients reporting a problem. Also check the Alerts and Product Recalls. Medical device registries are in the process of development in many countries. Can you find a few governmental agencies or health insurers that are beginning to establish such registries?

Information Technologies as Comparators

Health information technology is a broad term and encompasses electronic medical records, computerized provider order entry systems, remote monitoring, and communication technologies utilized to share information and impact services. Applications are broad. They may involve patient self-management with chronic conditions, shared decision making among providers and patients, and applications that promote wellness and health maintenance. Some technologies relate to medication monitoring and reminders, preventive service reminders, communications regarding laboratory and test results, adherence to treatment, assessment of problem lists, monitoring vital signs and health behaviors, and monitoring symptoms or adverse effects. As technology expands, so do the possible applications to promote health and improve functioning.

Comparative effectiveness research can provide an important mechanism from which to evaluate choices in health information technology. It is especially important with advancements in communication and the development of networks for the delivery of health services. Such advances have spawned subspecialties in medical care such as telehealth, telemedicine, telenursing, telepharmacy, and a range of other disciplines that utilize telecommunications for health-related purposes. The World Health Organization defined "eHealth" as the use of information

Explore
Check out some examples of Health Information Technology projects by searching for HealthIT AHRQ (http://healthit.ahrq.gov/). Funded projects are listed. Explore the range of projects underway. There is also an AHRQ Health IT YouTube channel where you can view some successful applications (https://www.youtube.com/ahrqhealthit). Also look at the International Society for Telemedicine & eHealth site (http://www.isfteh.org/). Check out the current projects in the Working Groups.

and communication technologies for health, and has several ongoing projects. Some governments call this HealthIT for Health Information Technology. Such applications can involve communication among health professionals, between patients and their providers, or among patients with other patients or lay caregivers. Commonly used devices such as cell phones and smartphones have found relevant uses. In some applications data are recorded on a device, stored, and transmitted at a later time (the store-and-forward or asynchronous approach). In other applications the data are shared in real time—also known as synchronous applications, such as videoconferencing.

There are extensive opportunities to evaluate the effectiveness of information technologies on people's health status and could involve patient-reported outcomes. Such applications can involve patient monitoring at home, the use of referral services, and the delivery of educational services to patients and families. It can involve the head-to-head comparison of two different electronic devices or of two different strategies. It could also involve a head-to-head comparison of a specific technology with a totally different approach (hi-tech versus low-tech) in various populations. Possibilities may involve complex processes over a period of time for chronic disease management, or incorporate time-specific therapy for episodic events which is delivered using technology. A critical element is its effect on an individual's health and functioning. In comparative effectiveness research, one would not just measure how well people adopt this technology, but how different technologies affect the patient's well-being or the health of a population as a whole.

Think
Think of all the electronic devices that you and your friends frequently use. Have you ever tried out health apps? Look online at some of more creative health apps available. Can you think of ways in which these may be applicable to improving health outcomes? List at least five possible applications.

Biologics as Comparators

Biologics are therapies derived from life forms—living or nonliving organisms and viruses. These include vaccines, allergenics, cellular and gene products, toxins and antitoxins, tissues, organs, blood and blood products, and xenotransplantation (the donation of nonhuman cells, tissues, and organs to human recipients). These include stem cell therapy and gene therapy. Such treatments can be as common as receiving an annual preventative flu shot, or as complex as a bilateral lung transplant in a patient with cystic fibrosis. There is a loose demarcation between biologics and drugs. Biologics are the products of living systems and are usually complex in structure while drugs are typically manufactured through chemical synthesis and have a well-defined structure. For some biologic products, the chemical composition is not fully known because they are mixtures of complex compounds and vary somewhat with the organism in which it was derived. For example, a unit of packed red blood cells utilized for transfusion is not a uniform entity as might be surmised at first glance. There are unique surface markers or antigens on red blood cells, even beyond those in the commonly recognized ABO and Rh blood groups. In fact, the blood group antigen gene mutation database (http://www.ncbi.nlm.nih.gov/projects/gv/rbc/xslcgi.fcgi?cmd=bgmut/summary) lists 34 blood group systems involving 44 genes and 1442 alleles (as of June 2013) with remarkable variation. What this means is that, unlike drugs which typically have a known specific chemical content, the transfusion given to one patient may be structurally quite different from the transfusion to another patient (or the same patient on a different day) because of different blood donors. This can present challenges in clinical research because the biologic intervention may not actually be a single intervention, but a series of somewhat-related interventions which could have differing effects in the recipients. This is true for many of the biologics, but not all. There are certain substances normally produced in humans that can be synthetically produced (e.g., insulin, glucagon, human growth hormone) and are structurally defined, which are regulated as drugs by the US Food and Drug Administration.

Human organ transplantation is a well-established therapy for certain patients with end-stage organ failure. Transplantation has been extensively utilized for patients with end-stage renal disease who receive kidney transplants, but is also used in patients who receive transplants of other organs such as heart, liver, lung, or pancreas. There are opportunities for comparative effectiveness research in this field—particularly as they relate to procedures and policies for donor procurement and approaches to more timely and effective receipt of the organs. And, as regenerative medicine advances in the future, there may be opportunities to compare allogeneic organ and tissue transfer with organ and tissue regeneration. The use of registries and large population-based databases with protracted longitudinal information can serve as resources for the evaluation of long-term effects.

Interestingly, the US Food and Drug Administration regulates biologics except for vascularized organ transplants such as kidney transplants, heart transplants, and liver transplants. The Health Resources Services Administration oversees such transplants in the United States, and it oversees bone marrow and cord blood donation as well.

Unlike most drugs, biologics tend to require special considerations regarding storage and administration. A significant proportion of medications can be taken orally, while many biologics require infusion or surgical procedures, and therefore health professionals may be necessary for administration. Such considerations regarding administration must be evaluated when planning a study.

Vaccines are common biologics that have been tested for effectiveness and safety. These include vaccines using live attenuated microorganisms such as those for measles, mumps, and rubella; inactivated microorganisms such as found in the polio vaccine; toxoid vaccines such as tetanus toxoids; protein subunit vaccines such as that for hepatitis B; and conjugate vaccines such as that for *Haemophilus influenzae* type B. Comparative effectiveness research can contribute to the study of vaccines by contrasting timing of administration, whether additional booster doses provide benefits, clarification of the types of individuals who would best benefit, and better definition of outcomes over time. For example, the use of large electronic databases of populations has yielded important investigations of vaccine safety using varied epidemiologic methods (Farrington, 2004).

Beyond vaccination, microorganisms have been investigated as therapy. One line of research has its origins in the ecology of the human microbiota. If you are not yet familiar with the research being conducted regarding the human microbiota, you should take a look (http://commonfund.nih.gov/hmp/). The discovery that we human beings are composites of life—that our structure and physiology are interconnected with microorganisms—has led to different perspectives regarding what is "normal" and possibilities for therapies. In fact, there are many more microbial cells in our bodies than there are human cells, and these microbes form a rich diversity of communities in the gastrointestinal tract, airways, urogenital tract, skin, and other sites. Researchers, with the help of molecular techniques, are now discovering how derangements in such normal microbial communities may be related to disease. One example of a potential therapy is that of fecal transplantation. Yes, that is indeed taking the feces of one person and inserting it into the intestinal tract of another person, which is sometimes done to hopefully change (for the better) the microbial communities that live there.

Gene therapy is another potential avenue for individuals with diseases that are the result of mutations in one or more genes. Gene therapy proposes to alter specific genes within the body either through introducing a new gene, inserting genes as replacements for mutated

Discover
Look at some of the microbiome sites. One example is the Human Microbiome Project (http://www.hmpdacc.org/). Check out the latest advances and news at this site, especially the impacts on health. Also check out the International Human Microbiome Consortium (http://www.human-microbiome.org/) and the Metagenomics of the Human Intestinal Tract (http://www.metahit.eu/). For some general overviews, you can visit one of the science news sites (Science Daily, EurekAlert!, NewScientist, etc.) and search for microbiome (referring to the collective genes of the microorganisms) or microbiota (referring to all microbes in a community at a particular time). Find anything interesting?

Explore
Stem cell therapy is another emergent therapeutic choice. Visit clinicaltrials.gov or the International Clinical Trials Registry Platform (ICTRP) and search for "stem cell." Look at the diversity of human trials underway to investigate various types of stem cell therapies. Can you find examples of trials that use autologous stem cells and studies that use allogeneic stem cells? Some of the sources of stem cells include the bone marrow, peripheral blood, and umbilical cord blood. Can you find examples of trials that use stem cells from these sources? Do you know of any stem cell therapies that are currently available for therapeutic use for specific diseases?

genes, or inactivating mutated genes. To deliver the genes to the targeted location, sometimes viruses or plasmids (small circular pieces of DNA that can replicate independently of the chromosome) are used. Various gene therapy studies are in progress. While not all initial human studies constitute comparative effectiveness research, ultimately one would expect that there would be examinations of whether such therapies compare favorably with other treatments to improve survival, functioning, and other patient-centered outcomes.

Surgical Procedures as Comparators

Surgery is a common procedure that has improved the lives of many people throughout the world. Surgical procedures are not regulated as are drugs or biologics for demonstration of safety and effectiveness prior to general use, although certain medical devices, which may be utilized in surgery, are regulated. Comparative effectiveness research may provide an important opportunity for contrasting different techniques and documenting associated patient outcomes. Does minimally invasive or keyhole surgery yield better patient outcomes than more invasive procedures? Does elective surgery in an outpatient surgical center yield similar effects as elective surgery in an acute care hospital? Topics for research may also include comparisons of various preoperative therapies, or may entail approaches to postdischarge management after inpatient surgery. Cross-disciplinary research may be valuable as well. How do patient outcomes compare after a specific surgical technique versus physical therapy for the same condition?

The National Surgical Quality Improvement Program has been on the forefront of evaluating the quality of surgical care in the United States (http://site.acsnsqip.org/). Within this program, measures were developed that reflect possible serious postsurgical complications such as blood clots, pneumonia, surgical site infection, urinary tract infection, renal failure, stroke, and cardiac arrest. The database generated from the collaborative efforts of team members in this program has yielded comparative studies that have influenced patient outcomes. Such studies are readily accessible within PubMed (search for National Surgical Quality Improvement Program).

Another example of a surgical initiative is the Safe Surgery Saves Lives program (http://www.who.int/patientsafety/safesurgery/en/). In a study conducted in various hospitals throughout the world, rates of complications and deaths decreased in surgical patients using a simple surgical

Take A Look
A copy of the World Health Organization Surgical Safety Checklist and its implementation manual is available online (http://www.who.int/patientsafety/safesurgery/ss_checklist/en/). Look at the documents at the WHO site and download a copy if you wish. Checklists are increasingly used in medicine as a safety tool. See if you can find other examples of safety-related checklists in medicine, nursing, pharmacy, and allied health fields.

safety checklist (Haynes, 2009). This included assessments at three time periods: sign-in (before induction of anesthesia), time out (before skin incision), and sign-out (before patient leaves the operating room). Since a considerable proportion of surgical complications are potentially preventable, this has been an important tool in improving care.

> **Explore**
> Visit the Cochrane Summaries site and type in "knee replacement surgery" in the search box at the top. Read the abstracts for several of these studies. Now search for whatever surgical procedure that is of particular interest to you. Did you learn anything new?

A readily available source for information regarding the effectiveness of different surgical procedures is the Cochrane Summaries site (http://summaries.cochrane.org/). This site contains information assembled by independent reviewers regarding randomized trials conducted throughout the world on various topics.

To obtain an overall view of the frequency of various surgical procedures, the Centers for Disease Control and Prevention has a webpage on Inpatient Surgery (http://www.cdc.gov/nchs/fastats/insurg.htm) which lists procedures by frequency (invasive and noninvasive procedures are combined). The Healthcare Cost and Utilization Project contains data regarding the Nationwide Inpatient Sample and procedures in the hospital setting are summarized (http://www.hcup-us.ahrq.gov/reports/statbriefs/sb_procedures.jsp). Various statistics regarding surgical procedures, as well as other procedures, are listed.

Screening Tests as Comparators

Screening tests constitute an important type of comparator. Screening, in medical and public health practice, refers to the **detection of a condition or disease before any symptoms are evident**. Often this involves a procedure or a laboratory test, the results of which are used to detect possible disease at a time when an individual does not notice any difference in their usual or normal functioning. This is in contrast to diagnostic tests, which are conducted when signs and symptoms of illness are readily apparent. Keep in mind that some terms used in medicine and public health have specific scientific meanings, but such terms are often used broadly by the general public. So when you visit media sites or public information sources, the word "screening" can be used broadly. But technically, screening has a narrower definition in medical research. Screening can be considered a part of secondary prevention initiatives in public health and preventive medicine. Primary prevention is conducted in the time period before the start of disease and is intended to prevent the incidence of disease. Secondary prevention is conducted after the initial stages of disease have begun but the individual does not yet recognize symptoms of the disease (e.g., screening). Tertiary prevention is conducted after the person is symptomatic and is intended to prevent complications after disease onset.

A screening test or procedure can be utilized as a comparator in comparative effectiveness research. For example, the effectiveness of screening for colorectal cancer may be assessed by evaluating several approaches such as the fecal occult blood test, sigmoidoscopy or colonoscopy. The researcher may also compare different screening schedules for the same test, such as annual versus biennial testing. Often it is important to test different screening timetables for people who are at higher baseline risk because of family history of disease than in people who are at lower risk. In such studies, the various screening regimens serve as the comparators and are linked to meaningful patient outcomes. Sometimes the outcomes relate to mortality. Do women who receive biennial mammograms live longer than women who do not adhere to this schedule? On a population basis, are there more healthy years of life (better functioning, less disability) associated with one screening strategy versus another?

Evaluation of screening may involve using a randomized controlled trial design. Individuals may be randomized to one screening regimen versus another, and are observed for mortality or severe disability generally over a protracted period of time. Needless to say, these studies take time and are relatively expensive to conduct. Sometimes there is information from entire populations, some of whom received one screening test and some who received another. Such large databases with extensive longitudinal information can also be useful in providing information, although it may be difficult to sort out whether the results are due to the real differences in the screening regimens or differences in the underlying characteristics of the people who chose one regimen over another.

You have probably already had a screening test. Newborn screening for congenital and genetic disorders such as phenylketonuria, hypothyroidism, and sickle cell disease is common. In elementary school, children may be screened for vision and hearing. Almost every time an adult has a clinic visit, blood pressure is measured which screens for hypertension in those without such pre-existing diagnosis. A list of various preventive screening measures (www.uspreventiveservicestaskforce.org/) can be found at the US Preventive Services Task Force site.

Discover
Discover screening tests which have been reviewed based on scientific evidence. Find six screening tests for the early disease detection in adults (http://www.uspreventiveservicestaskforce.org/adultrec.htm) and six screening tests for children or adolescents (http://www.uspreventiveservicestaskforce.org/tfchildcat.htm). What types of conditions are most often associated with screening? These current screening recommendations are based on evidence from medical research studies. After reviewing these recommendations, are there any other screening tests that you think would be important to review but are not yet on this list? If so, you have the opportunity to suggest this topic and submit it to the Task Force (http://www.uspreventiveservicestaskforce.org/uspstf_NewTopic/).

Diet and Food as Comparators

Food and beverages are arguably the most important therapies for life. Without them, you die. The types and quantities of foods and beverages as well as the timing of meals impact the functioning of all your cells in your body as well as your normal microbiota. These everyday dietary choices critically impact how your body functions. They impact how you feel, how you move, and how you think.

It is not uncommon to overlook this type of "therapy" because food (and I'll include liquid food, beverages, in this definition as well) is not usually something administered by a health professional. You don't have to visit a doctor, dentist, or therapist to obtain food. It's all there for the taking at grocery stores, in the garden, and at restaurants. Its' importance can be overlooked, but shouldn't be.

Dietary choices can be important comparators utilized in research studies. Structuring such dietary interventions can, however, be a challenge. Just try to go through the mental exercise of devising a study whereby some people would be eating certain foods while other people would be eating something else. Imagine the problems associated with, first, cajoling people to eat what you want them to, being able to monitor whether they actually did it, and seeing a noticeable result in a reasonable amount of time (remember, it's not likely that your study will last ten years).

> **Try This**
> Make a preliminary attempt at designing a dietary study using food (not dietary supplements but actual food items or a variety of foods) and choose a meaningful outcome that would be important to most people. Make a list of six items that may need to be considered in order to do this research.

Listed below are some approaches that investigators have used in research studies in order to record dietary intake:

- **Food records.** Basically, a person records all the food and beverages he or she eats throughout the day (and night when appropriate). Details can be given regarding specific brands and recipes. Sometimes the person is asked to weigh the foods before eating and subtract remaining food not eaten. This is generally done for several days with both weekday and weekend information.
- **24-hour dietary recall.** A person is asked to recall all the food and beverages that he/she ate or drank during a particular 24-hour period. Sometimes recall of several 24-hour periods are requested, with both weekday and weekend information. An example is the automated multiple-pass 24-hour recall, which is a computer-enhanced approach for multiple-day dietary collection using either an in-person or phone interviewer. The multiple passes are mechanisms inbuilt to probe and revisit information during the process.

- **Food frequency questionnaire.** A person is given a questionnaire with lists of foods and beverages and is asked to record how often he or she ate these items. The person is often asked to record their usual intake and generally is given a specific time period for this intake, such as within the last year or within the last month.
- **Population differences in diets.** Knowledge of the types of diets used by different populations (often by geographic region or by cultural/ethnic practices) may be utilized for research purposes. The Mediterranean diet would be an example.

There is a wealth of information regarding methodology for each of the above approaches, and there have been instruments developed for each method. There are also permutations of the approaches listed above. So, instead of a person filling out a questionnaire, it could be an interviewer who asks the questions. Some of the instruments may be electronic and can be completed online. Dietitians are experts in this field, so if you are planning a dietary study, inclusion of a dietitian would be wise.

Check It Out
Look at the types of dietary information routinely collected by the National Health and Nutrition Study (NHANES), which is located at the Centers for Disease Control and Prevention (CDC) site. They collect data regarding dietary behavior, 24-hour dietary recall, and food frequency questionnaires. Note that the NHANES provides its data free online to researchers, so you can read through the questionnaires and download the actual data. Many researchers have used the NHANES to publish dietary studies. Go to PubMed online and search for NHANES. Do you see some studies utilizing this national survey?

There are some areas of clinical research in which diet has been a critical component for many years. Obstetrics and pediatrics are examples. Dietary interventions have been important aspects of research in pregnancy, during the postnatal period (breastfeeding, infant formulas), throughout childhood, and into adolescence. Diet has been recognized as an essential component of normal growth and as such, nutritional interventions during these periods have been examined. Because of developmental differences in cognition and memory, often different methods for data collection are necessary. For example, in young children, weighed food records may require the help of parents or caregivers.

Dietary research has also been important in developing countries or in areas in which food scarcity is a problem. Studies in children and pregnant women, in particular, have been of interest. In many studies, the dietary interventions were administered at the person level and, in other studies, the intervention involved implementation of a national or regional dietary policy. Mechanisms to assess food intake should take into account the particular cultural context of the region. Food practices and preferences vary greatly by culture and therefore, it is important to recognize these elements by collaborating with local individuals who have expertise in practices.

Dietary research has also been important in studies of chronic disease such as cancer. The Risk Factor Monitoring and Methods Branch of the National

Cancer Institute developed methods to assess usual dietary intake. The NCI Diet History Questionnaire has been freely available for years (http://riskfactor.cancer.gov/dhq2/). This questionnaire may be useful for baseline information regarding dietary intake in comparative effectiveness research studies. Also available from the National Cancer Institute is the Automated Self-administered 24-hour Recall (ASA24). It is a Web-based tool that enables the study participants to self-administer 24-hour dietary recalls (http://riskfactor.cancer.gov/tools/instruments/asa24/). Use of the tool is free for researchers and methods for study management and data analyses are available. There is a version for adults, as well as one for children. The recall can be administered in either English or Spanish.

Download
Search for Diet History Questionnaire and National Cancer Insitute (http://riskfactor.cancer.gov/dhq2/). There are free paper-based forms and web-based entry for this questionnaire, as well as software for analyses. You can download the forms and software if you wish and try it out. Also visit the NCI ASA24 Automated Self-administered 24-hour Recall site (http://riskfactor.cancer.gov/tools/instruments/asa24/). Look at the information available to see whether you may be interested in using these tools within a research study. While at this site, you may also want to look at the main Risk Factor Monitoring and Methods section on Tools for Researchers (http://riskfactor.cancer.gov/). There are additional tools that may be of interest to you.

There are certain universities in which dietary methods have been extensively developed due to the interest and research experience of the faculty. Examples include the University of Illinois with its online Nutrition Analysis Tool (NAT), the University of Minnesota Nutrition Data System for Research (complete system available for research at a fee), and the Iowa State University software for dietary intake (http://www.side.stat.iastate.edu/).

Not only is diet important for people in their daily lives at home and work, but nutritional therapy can be crucial in the context of hospital medicine and for residents of skilled nursing facilities. Patients with metabolic disorders, gastrointestinal disease, immune disorders, renal disease, and patients undergoing surgery have particular nutritional needs. Comparisons of different therapeutic approaches can be an important aspect of improving patient outcomes. Total parenteral nutrition and enteral feeding have both been evaluated as comparators in specific situations. The types of formulas utilized in such feeding regimens are important to be evaluated. Also, routes of delivery and management of care are also possibilities for comparators in research.

Discover
Want to explore what is in your food? The United States Department of Agriculture (USDA) houses online databases on food content (http://ndb.nal.usda.gov/). Click on a food and see what it contains! Also look at the variety of different food-related databases available. There are databases for micronutrients, macronutrients, phytochemicals, vitamins, and minerals. Try out their "Fat Intake Screener" or their "Healthy Body Calculator" (http://fnic.nal.usda.gov/dietary-guidance/dietary-assessment). The "SuperTracker" for tracking nutrition and physical activity has the potential for incorporation into comparative effectiveness research studies (https://www.supertracker.usda.gov/default.aspx).

Exercise and Mobility as Comparators

Evaluation of exercise regimens can serve as viable options in comparative effectiveness research. This may include specific programs in aerobic exercise, step training, or resistance training. It may involve a simple intervention to increase walking distance by using pedometers, or may include swimming or water exercises. There are particular exercises associated to improve balance, flexibility, or strength. For patients who are in recovery and are undergoing rehabilitation, a comparative study by a physical therapist could be valuable. There may also be interventions that are meant to improve adherence to habitual exercise regimens.

While physical activity may serve as a comparator in a trial or longitudinal study, there may also be instances in which the patient-centered outcome of the research study is an improvement in mobility. That is, in some comparative effectiveness studies, physical activity serves as one of the therapies under investigation, while in other studies, changes in physical activity (functional mobility) serve as the outcome. This is an example whereby a given behavior (physical activity) can be used as different elements within study design.

There are mobility interventions that combine movement with entertainment, an example being dance. Such interventions that interweave several objectives may be important to evaluate. That is, dance often includes an added social component. There are other movement exercises such as tai chi that may constitute suitable comparators for some investigations. There are many creative interactive body-movement video games that integrate competitive entertainment with exercise. Such games can involve people across various ages, from young to old, particularly since there are motion-sensing games that circumvent the need for manual controllers. Of course, there are a wide variety of sports that can constitute interventions or therapies and also are fun, provide social engagement, and encourage movement at the same time. Not all need be relegated to the highly talented athlete. While one might think that such studies may not be necessary because we know that these activities tend to be beneficial, there are times when a specific physical activity regimen may warrant investigation. Standardized questionnaires of walking and bicycling available for researchers are given at the National Cancer Institute (http://appliedresearch.cancer.gov/tools/paq/).

From a wider perspective, interventions that involve restructuring of the environment, often called the "built environment," include configuration of human-made structures and

Think
What types of physical activity could be utilized for a wide range of ages? Name at least five comparators that incorporate physical activity which may be feasible for studies which enroll individuals who are overweight. Can you find some published scientific studies demonstrating that physical activity improved health outcomes? What types of outcomes were improved?

the surrounding spaces so as to affect livability and activity levels. Such built environments may improve walkability or bikability or access to green spaces. Therefore, a population-based intervention can be the restructuring of such human environments to encourage physical mobility in the community as a whole.

Psychotherapeutic and Social Approaches as Comparators

Psychotherapy is an umbrella term for a number of different interpersonal approaches which involve the collaboration between patients and practitioners, and which assist individuals with problems or issues related to mental health. Cognitive interventions, specific behavioral approaches, interpersonal therapy, and psychodynamic therapies are conventional treatments. There are also combinations of such therapies. The types of psychotherapeutic approaches are quite varied and may involve talking with a psychiatrist, psychologist, or mental health worker. An example is a therapy called Seeking Safety which is a treatment that has been used for individuals who have experienced posttraumatic stress disorder, trauma, or substance abuse. This treatment involves a combination of cognitive, behavioral, and interpersonal techniques. Many of the psychotherapeutic therapies involve setting goals and resolving issues through communication, adaptations in behavior, and cognitive exercises. Therapy may be administered to individuals, couples, families, or other groups.

Cognitive behavioral therapy provides a mechanism by which patients achieve a better understanding of, and can influence reactions to, their thoughts and feelings. It has been utilized with conditions such as anxiety, depression, insomnia, chemical addictions, anger management, and phobias.

Behavioral therapeutic approaches may serve as suitable interventions within the context of comparative effectiveness research. For example, such therapy may involve head-to-head comparisons of techniques meant to change perceived negative behaviors such as suicidal thoughts, or to overcome phobias. Other comparisons may have the intent to increase positive family relations through various types of counseling. Other approaches may be to improve the psyche or to have calming effects, such as music therapy. Hypnosis has been utilized for a variety of conditions such as pain or gastrointestinal problems. Other comparators of interest may involve internal cognitive techniques and include meditation, stress reduction approaches, and mindfulness. For conditions such as eating disorders, anxiety, depression, posttraumatic stress disorder, and other disorders with a behavioral component, comparative studies can be designed to evaluate the impact of alternative approaches on meaningful outcomes.

Therapies that speak to the connections between people may have a significant impact on functioning. Humans are social creatures. Family and community can provide support that impacts one's ability to recognize disorders, seek medical attention when appropriate, secure access to transportation for medical services, provide support during hospital stays and when under active treatment therapies, and conduct day-to-day nursing activities after one is discharged from the hospital. Aspects of social support can be measured and utilized as comparators in studies of patient outcomes. The social support might be a simple peer-support system, the presence of a health buddy or friend, or the presence of a wide network of support. Other aspects of our social environments may also be of interest. Do activities associated with more human interaction impact health-related outcomes? Such questions can be answered by using comparative effectiveness research.

While often we think of social support for the needs of a patient (as a recipient), another valid comparator are individuals acting as givers. For example, is volunteering associated with better health outcomes? Does the type of volunteering make a difference? The reasoning behind this avenue of investigation is that having a sense of purpose and doing something for others may possibly have health benefits for recipients and volunteers.

Discover

Visit PLOS Medicine to find a study entitled, "Comparative Efficacy of Seven Psychotherapeutic Interventions for Patients with Depression: A Network Meta-Analysis" (PLoS Med. 2013;10(5):e1001454). The authors compared seven therapies for their effects on depression symptoms after treatment. Read through how and what types of studies were selected. Which therapy or therapies showed benefits in reducing symptoms of depression?

Delivery Systems as Comparators

One of the aspects of health care that is of direct import to patients is its delivery. Listen to people as they talk about their everyday experiences: "I took off of work so I could have a blood test. Had to wait two hours until they could fit me in. The lady took my blood but didn't know what it was for. I asked if I could see my results and was told no—they couldn't release them without permission. To this day, I don't know what that test was all about and don't know the results. I just know that I lost a half day of work."

Health care delivery relates to how services are received by patients. Delivery system research can encompass a wide net of interventions that relate to the structure of health care, the processes within that structure, and the coordination and interactions among these elements. From a patient-centered approach, the coordination of these systems and the methods of delivery can be of great importance in everyday life.

Health care delivery systems, in general, vary greatly from country to country and, in the United States, from state to state. There can also be significant variability of delivery in the same region, based upon the characteristics and resources of the providers and those of the patients. From a research perspective, international or regional differences in delivery systems can provide an opportunity to investigate meaningful outcomes. Disparities between health care services received by different types of people may provide an occasion to conduct comparative effectiveness research. While occasionally differences may be due to limited access to certain services, it may be worthwhile to investigate whether there are barriers to delivery that could be ameliorated through various interventions. In other situations there may an imbalance among the personnel available, or the lack of systems in place for communication. Head-to-head comparisons of several approaches and direct measurement of outcomes relevant to patients are important in comparative effectiveness research.

Specific health care policies can be utilized as comparators. Great impacts in the health of societies can sometimes be seen with the enactment of national policies that affect the health of entire populations. It may be a preventive initiative, policies regarding the availability or access to certain drugs, or policies that affect the delivery of care. A change in payment for a health service or a change in access to certain services due to enactment of a new law at the local, state, or federal level can serve as a comparator for patient outcome research. Comparisons can be made between what occurred prior to the policy versus what occurred in the post-policy period. Alternatively, contrasts in patient outcomes can be made between a segment of the population in which the policy was enacted and a different segment of population unaffected by the policy during a concurrent time period. Of note in the United States, the implementation of the Patient Protection and Affordable Care Act can serve as a basis to compare outcomes before and after the policies were enacted, as well as differences between health care delivery systems from state to state.

Discover

In the United States, the health care delivery system is undergoing change with the enactment of the Patient Protection and Affordable Care Act. Go to the US Department of Health and Human Services site (and other sites) to look for information regarding this Act and notable changes in services that are underway. Search for "Health Insurance Marketplace." What are the features of this Marketplace? What are the "essential health benefits" within this Marketplace? Look at the Marketplace in several states and compare differences. Such differences can form the underlying source for comparative effectiveness research studies. What is a Collaborative Care Network and what is the purpose of such networks? What is an Accountable Care Organization and what is the purpose of such organizations? What is a Medical Home and what is the purpose of Medical Homes? What is Value Based Purchasing and what is its purpose? How does this differ from Fee-for-Service? What impacts do you think such entities will have on patient outcomes and the health of people nationwide?

Comparators and Adherence

People have minds of their own. Even when they choose a specific therapy, they might do it for awhile but then stop. Or they may say they plan to use a particular regimen but they don't. From a research perspective, there are several elements in play here. One relates to the effectiveness of one regimen versus another. The other element relates to adherence to a regimen. In comparative effectiveness research, the investigators can use both of these elements (effectiveness and adherence) in evaluating health options (Chubak, 2013). It is possible to have a regimen that is more effective than another, but because of difficulties with access to health services or dislike of the procedure, adherence is low. In this instance, the less effective regimen might actually provide more healthy years of life in the population as a whole because more people adhere to it. In such instances, it may be possible to conduct additional comparative effectiveness research just to address the adherence issues such as comparing methods to increase accessibility to the effective therapy. However, there may be select instances in which feasibility, acceptability, and other relevant issues may play a more significant role than effectiveness alone.

Other Comparators

There are a variety of other comparators available for investigators. For example, a device need not be a designated medical device, but something rather common in ordinary life. Researchers have used shoes as comparators. Proper fitting shoes are very important because of underlying risks posed by advanced diabetes mellitus or peripheral vascular disease. Other clothing items may constitute an intervention in a research study, such as clothing that reduces ultraviolet radiation or clothing that cools instead of heats the body. A very old-fashioned therapy is heat (or cold) therapy. Heating pads for specific conditions and ice packs for others have been used for many years. The evaluation of when to use these therapies and for how long would be a natural choice for a comparator in research.

There can be nonhuman comparators. Some of our best companions—pets—sometimes are trained in simple tasks. This can become the basis of an intervention. In other instances, the pets may not be trained at all, but serve psychological needs as a companion or could serve as an impetus for better health behaviors (e.g., cardiovascular effects of dog walking). One can use comparators that are typically present during people's usual everyday lives.

Discover

See if you can find other types of comparators which are not listed here. Think of other activities, behaviors, or therapies that relate to health that have not been specifically mentioned, yet could be candidates as a comparator in a research study. Note that some of the US National Priority Topics in comparative effectiveness research are quite broad. Sometimes the selection of the comparators is left to the investigators. For example, one of the priorities is to "compare the effectiveness of different strategies to engage and retain patients in care and to delineate barriers to care, especially for members of populations that experience health disparities." Another is to "compare the effectiveness of different treatment strategies on the frequency and lost productivity in people with chronic, frequent migraine headaches."

Education is frequently used as a comparator—not specifically in most clinical studies but surely in educational research. In terms of health research, education is often used in the hopes that it will translate to behavioral change (of patients and/or providers). Education regarding a specific procedure or therapy can be used as a comparator or, alternatively, education may be one of several components of a larger multicomponent therapy. In usual practice, it is often difficult to separate educational aspects of therapy because clinicians often give instructions when administering therapies. However, when purposely utilized, the medium can be very narrow—specifically targeted to certain patients—or very broad, such as a YouTube video, a television commercial, or a billboard announcement. Educational interventions are often used in public health.

Keep an open mind. If there are other types of possible techniques or approaches that may impact health or functioning, they may well be candidates for comparative effectiveness research.

4

The Effect

Conceptualization of the effects of treatment begins with an examination of health. What is good health? How would this be defined? The World Health Organization defines good health as a state of complete physical, social, and mental well-being, and not merely the absence of disease or infirmity. So this definition recognizes three important entities—physical status, social connections, and mental health.

The purpose of comparative effectiveness research is to provide information regarding the effectiveness of interventions or services. The word "effectiveness" relates to the outcome—the effect of the intervention. The researcher is essentially asking, "Of the interventions tested, which one did a better job in making people healthier? Did the interventions improve physical status, social connections, and/or mental health?"

Think
If you were to define good health, what would your definition be?

Outcomes have been extensively researched in various disciplines so you will find different names for an outcome in the biomedical literature. These include:

- Effect
- Endpoint
- Result
- Consequence
- Response
- Dependent variable

In terms of planning a study, an examination of the outcome is one of the first steps after the general research question or hypothesis has been posed. What specific outcomes should we use? How should these outcomes be measured? How have these outcomes been assessed in previous research?

The types of outcomes studied in comparative effectiveness research fall into several broad categories. The first category includes outcomes that deal with the health status of individuals and, in particular, with potential beneficial effects of one intervention versus another. Such outcomes are generally the primary endpoints in comparative effectiveness research. They are the results that one would hope to achieve: Greater mobility. Less pain. Effortless breathing. Better sight. Another category includes studies in which the focus is more on the adverse effects of interventions. For example, after a drug is found to be efficacious, it is marketed and may be prescribed to patients throughout the country. Sometimes there may be unexpected adverse effects of therapies when given to large numbers of people, due to either yet unrecognized characteristics of individuals who may not respond well to such therapy or low background rates of adverse events associated with the therapy itself. Comparative effectiveness research can provide information on these effects and the subgroups of people who may be at particular risk.

Patient-Reported Outcomes

A hallmark of comparative effectiveness research is the intentional use of patient-reported outcomes whenever possible. Patient-reported outcomes are observations by patients related to their well-being. These are directly stated by the patient and are not interpreted or inferred through a clinician or another person. Thus, they constitute any report of a patient's health status, experience, or behavior that comes directly from the patient without interpretation by anyone else. Measures can be reported such as the degree of pain severity, or changes in affect can be conveyed such as feeling better now compared to last week. Often these are symptoms, but not necessarily. While symptoms often relate to observations related to illness or disorders, patient-reported outcomes also encompass observations related to wellness, functioning, satisfaction, perceptions, level of understanding or agreement. Both "I've never felt happier in my life" and "I am so sad and down—I can barely drag myself out of bed" are patient reports that can serve as a foundation for a patient-reported outcome. Alternatively, the researcher may use a visual analogue scale whereby happiness and sadness are at opposite extremes and the participants record their mood at specified times during the course of the study. There are also visual analogue scales for pain whereby the patient can report the intensity of their pain along a gradient. General categories of measurements for responses include the following:

- **Visual analog scale.** Pictorial representation of extremes with a mechanism for subject response along the scale.
- **Pictorial response.** Pictures meant to represent symptoms, feelings, or other entities are selected by respondents. Not necessarily on a scale of extremes.
- **Likert scale.** Ordered set of responses presented in a gradation.
- **Checklist.** List of questions or items requiring a check or short response.

- **Rating scale.** Categories of items that are numbered for respondent choice regarding degree of quality or like/dislike.
- **Record, diary, or blog.** Respondent records items as they occur in real time.

> **Explore**
> Look at the appearance of various visual analogue scales for pain. That is, use your favorite online search engine and type in "visual analogue scale for pain" in the Images section. Do you have any favorites?

While there are some patient-reported outcomes that have been utilized in clinical research for many decades, there are others that are not frequently seen in the context of research. Therefore, development of relevant measures may be necessary prior to the study. Development of such measures is a process that involves exploration of the types of outcomes that are of importance to patients with specific conditions, taking into account their age and personal characteristics that may impact preferences. Sometimes this involves conducting a pre-study survey of patients with a specific disorder in order to obtain their opinions regarding expectations of the risks and benefits of possible therapies. Sometimes this involves focus groups of people with specific conditions (e.g., chronic heart failure) and an exploration of patients' typical functioning and experiences in daily life.

> **Try This**
> Start thinking about patient-reported outcomes from your perspective. Make a list of five outcomes that would be most desirable to you in terms of your health. What outcomes are very important to your physical, social, and mental well-being? Begin to explore how you could possibly measure these outcomes.

In various research studies, there are some routinely used symptom checklists that reflect an underlying construct that may be helpful in measuring outcomes. If you have never seen such checklists before, it is informative to look at some examples. Below is an example of the Patient Health Questionnaire depression module 9 (PHQ-9). It contains nine questions that measure depression severity.

- Over the *last two weeks*, how often have you been bothered by any of the following problems?
    - Little interest or pleasure in doing things.
    - Feeling down, depressed, or hopeless.
    - Trouble falling or staying asleep, or sleeping too much.
    - Feeling tired or having little energy.
    - Poor appetite or overeating.
    - Feeling bad about yourself—or that you are a failure or have let yourself or your family down.
    - Trouble concentrating on things, such as reading the newspaper or watching television.
    - Moving or speaking so slowly that other people could have noticed? Or the opposite—being so fidgety or restless that you have been moving around a lot more than usual.

¤ Thoughts that you would be better off dead or of hurting yourself in some way.

For each of these nine instances, the person answers regarding the frequency of occurrence: "Not at all," "Several days," "More than half the days," or "Nearly every day." In terms of a comparative effectiveness research study, an investigator could administer this questionnaire before and after administration of the therapies. This could allow the researcher to compare the pre–post differences in scores on this questionnaire, as well as the difference in scores between the various comparators under investigation.

There are instruments or assessments that capture quality of life, functioning, activities of daily living, and pain that are commonly used by health professionals. Sometimes such instruments are collectively labeled as health-related quality of life measures. There are several domains, including physical, functional, psychological/emotional, and social/occupational. However, not all measures include each of these domains. Some commonly used instruments are:

¤ **Basic activities of daily living (basic ADLs or BADLs)**. These are assessments of whether the person can take care of oneself with regard to dressing, eating, ambulating, toileting and hygiene.
¤ **Instrumental activities of daily living (IADLs)**. These are assessments of whether the person can function independently in caring for oneself. These activities include shopping, housekeeping, accounting, food preparation, medication use, communication, and transportation. There are occasional variations in the types of activities measured; some scales include the ability to respond to emergencies, taking care of others, taking care of pets, and other behaviors.
¤ **The Barthel Index**. This index measures mobility and ability to perform personal care.
¤ For children, there are many **developmental scales and instruments** used to assess whether a child is functioning at their age-expected level (e.g., Battelle Developmental Inventory Screening Test, Denver Developmental Screening Test). Some of the scales deal with language, others with cognitive abilities and problem solving, physical and motor skills, or social and emotional behavior. There are specific quality of life instruments for children with chronic illness such as cancer (e.g., Children's Adjustment to Cancer Index), type 1 diabetes (e.g., Pediatric Quality of Life Inventory Type 1 Diabetes Module), and asthma (e.g., Paediatric Asthma Quality of Life Questionnaire).
¤ **EUROQol.** This is a standardized instrument for measuring health-related quality of life. It includes mobility, self-care, usual activities, pain/discomfort, anxiety/depression, health state.

- **Health Utilities Index.** This standardized instrument measures health status and quality of life in patients, as well as produces utility scores. It encompasses a family of health profiles and assigns a value to the quality of life, taking into account function, impairments, perceptions, and social factors.
- **Health and Activities Limitations Index.** This index measures perceived health and limitations of activities. It originated from items on the National Health Interview Survey.
- **Quality of Well-Being Scale.** This scale includes reference-weighted measures of symptoms and functioning. It includes mobility, physical activity, and social activity.
- **Visual Functioning Questionnaire (VFQ-25).** This questionnaire, from the National Eye Institute, contains questions regarding vision and eye health.
- **Functional Assessment of Chronic Illness Therapy.** This assessment refers to a collection of questionnaires related to the quality of life for patients with chronic illnesses. It includes physical, social/family, emotional, and functional well-being.

The 36-Item Short Form Health Survey (SF-36) was developed as a part of the Medical Outcomes Study and is a common instrument for assessing functioning, well-being, and health-related quality of life. It includes general health, change in health, physical functioning, pain, emotional functioning, social functioning, and mental health. For example, four of the items on the survey are as follows:

During the past four weeks, have you had any of the following problems with your work or other regular daily activities as a result of your physical health?

- Cut down the amount of time you spent on work or other activities.
- Accomplished less than you would like.
- Were limited in the kind of work or other activities.
- Had difficulty performing the work or other activities (for example, it took extra effort).

Check It Out
The RAND Corporation developed the SF-36 and it is available online (http://www.rand.org/health/surveys_tools/mos/mos_core_36item.html). The instrument can be downloaded, as well as the instructions for scoring. You might also want to check out their Surveys & Tools section (http://www.rand.org/health/surveys_tools.html), which lists several instruments for various populations, including other quality of life surveys.

There are quality of life assessments for children and adolescents as well. The Pediatric Quality of Life Inventory is age-specific. For example, some of the health and activity questions for school-aged children (ages 8–12 years) are:

1. It is hard for me to walk more than one block.
2. It is hard for me to run.

3. It is hard for me to do sports activity or exercise.
4. It is hard for me to lift something heavy.
5. It is hard for me to take a bath or shower by myself.
6. It is hard for me to do chores around the house.
7. I hurt or ache.
8. I have low energy.

The answers are scored on a Likert scale of Never, Almost never, Sometimes, Often, and Almost always.

There are also patient-reported outcomes that are utilized in real-time assessment for immediate feedback (www.nihpromis.org/) such as before and after treatment sessions. These approaches are sometimes used in mental health settings, but there may be other applications as well. For example, the Outcome Rating Scale has the following questions:

> I'm going to ask some questions about four different areas of your life, including your individual, interpersonal, and social functioning. Each of these questions is based on a 1 to 10 scale, with 10 being high (or very good) and 1 being low (or very bad). Thinking back over the last week (or since our last conversation), how would you rate:
>
> 1. How you have been doing personally? (on the scale from 1 to 10)
> 2. How have things been going in your relationships? (on the scale from 1 to 10)
> 3. How have things been going for you socially? (on the scale from 1 to 10)
> 4. So, given your answers on these specific areas of your life, how would you rate how things are in your life overall?

The Session Rating Scale has the following questions:

> I'm going to ask some questions about our session today, including how well you felt understood, the degree to which we focused on what you wanted to talk about, and whether our work together was a good fit. Each of these questions is based on a 1 to 10 scale, with 10 being high (or very good) and 1 being low (or very bad).
>
> Thinking back over our conversation, how would you rate:
>
> 1. On a scale of 1–10, to what degree did you feel heard and understood today, 10 being completely and 1 being not at all?
> 2. On a scale of 1–10, to what degree did we work on the issues that you wanted to work on today, 10 being completely and 1 being not at all?
> 3. On a scale of 1–10, how well did my approach, the way I worked, make sense and fit for you?
> 4. So, given your answers on these specific areas, how would you rate how things were in today's session overall, with 10 meaning that the session was right for you and 1 meaning that something important that was missing from the visit?

The International Society for Quality of Life Research provides an online users guide to implementing patient-reported outcomes assessment (Snyder, 2012). This may be helpful for a general overview. A pdf of the document is freely available online (http://www.isoqol.org/research/isoqol-publications). There is also general information regarding health-related quality of life research and the methods by which measures are developed.

Patient-Reported Outcomes Measurement Information System

There have been national efforts to standardize the types of questions that are meant to capture patient-reported outcomes. Often there is variation in the ways in which questions are asked. It is important that the questions themselves are valid and reliable. That is, they should accurately measure what they are intended to measure and show comparable results with repeated testing. In addition, it can be useful to examine a broad range of questions that are applicable to patients across the various types of issues relevant to health and functioning. It is also valuable when the items are tested in diverse groups of people—by age, gender, race, health conditions, and other factors relevant to the intended participants. Different formats are available for administration. These would go beyond just a series of questions on paper and may include computer adaptive testing (CAT) or other forms of input. One such Patient Reported Outcomes Measurement Information System is funded by the National Institutes of Health. Adult banks of questions include the following domains: anger, anxiety, depression, fatigue, pain behavior, pain interference, physical function, satisfaction with discretionary social interactions, satisfaction with social roles, sleep disturbance, wake disturbance, and global health.

Check It Out
Search online for PROMIS or Patient Reported Outcomes Measurement Information System (www.nihpromis.org). Go to Measures and look at some of the sample questions. For example, one of the questions is: In the past seven days...
¤ I have trouble starting things because I am tired.
  ¤ Not at all
  ¤ A little bit
  ¤ Somewhat
  ¤ Quite a bit
  ¤ Very much

Look at the range of questions. They include physical health, anxiety, depression, fatigue, sleep disturbance, social function, pain interference, and global health. Notice that you can request a zip file of the PROMIS short forms and it will be emailed to you. Try it out. Also, if you select Software Demonstration, you can fill out some questions online. Go ahead and do this. Look at the type of output that you receive at the end.

From a researcher's point of view, the PROMIS site is practical. The questions are readily available and have been tested and validated. Additional questions will be available over time.

There are other agencies and organizations that develop Patient-Reported Outcomes (called PRO) and Patient-Reported Outcome Measures (called PROM). One such group is the MAPI Research Trust, which houses a

Patient-Reported Outcome and Quality of Life Instruments Database (http://www.proqolid.org/). The MAPI Research Trust (http://www.mapi-trust.org) allows open access to the following types of instruments that are useful in comparative effectiveness research:

- Health-related quality of life
- Health-related quality of end of life
- Patient satisfaction (for a wide range of health-related entities)
- Physical functioning (limitations and restrictions)
- Psychological functioning (affect and cognitive measures)
- Signs and symptoms (physical and psychological)
- Social functioning (work, school, community)
- Adherence to treatment
- Utilities (these are summary measures used by certain researchers to quantify the quality of life)

The MAPI Research Trust is a nonprofit organization dedicated to education, information, and dissemination of patient-reported outcomes and epidemiology. They include a network of over 3,000 researchers worldwide and distribute over 110 questionnaires. Of note, translations are available for some questionnaires. They also house databases such as RefPRO, which is a bibliographic database on patient-reported outcomes and epidemiology. PROQOLID is their Patient-Reported Outcome and Quality of Life Instruments Database, which is an excellent resource for comparative effectiveness researchers. The methods of administration for the instruments available via the Patient-Reported Outcome and Quality of Life Instruments Database are quite varied, and include various electronic options and choice of different administrators. The MAPI Research Trust also houses PROLabels that contains data regarding drugs approved with patient-reported outcome labeling claims. Drugs must satisfy specific criteria regarding claims prior to placement on the drug labels. Therefore, drug regulatory agencies in various countries have also been working to standardize patient-reported outcomes.

Another source for standardized patient-reported outcomes is through the Critical Path Institute, which is working with the US Food and Drug Administration. They formed a Patient-Reported Outcome Consortium (http://c-path.org/PRO.cfm), which works to

Check It Out
Go to the Patient-Reported Outcome and Quality of Life Instruments Database (PROQOLID) site (http://www.proqolid.org/). When at the site, search for any topic that is of interest to you. You can also browse the instruments or questionnaires. Click on one of the instruments. Usually, at the bottom are references to the scientific publications for this particular instrument. In addition, sometimes there is a link to a website specifically for this instrument. If you are a student and do not yet have funds for using this instrument in a research study, you may be able to obtain a copy of some instruments through their catalog (under Questionnaire Licensing, select Our Catalog) and filling out a limited use agreement. Or sometimes, a copy of the instrument is available as an appendix in scientific journal articles.

develop valid instruments for research in particular areas such as rheumatoid arthritis, depression, cognition, irritable bowel syndrome, and asthma. They also developed an Electronic Patient-Reported Outcome (ePRO) Consortium (http://c-path.org/ePRO.cfm). Their intent is to develop patient-reported outcome measures to be utilized in clinical trials.

Patient-reported outcome measures are routinely and openly reported in some countries. In the United Kingdom, such measures are available for patients undergoing certain medical procedures. Take a look at some of these online if you wish (type in "patient-reported outcome measures UK" or go to http://www.hscic.gov.uk/proms). Patient-reported outcome measures have been collected since 2009 by providers in the National Health Service and are available for patients undergoing hip and knee replacements, and hernias and varicose vein procedures.

In the United States, the Agency for Healthcare Research and Quality houses a National Quality Measure Clearinghouse (http://www.qualitymeasures.ahrq.gov/index.aspx). It lists publications in which various patient-relevant measures were used, some of which are patient reported. There are also sections on selecting measures, the validity of measures, and comparing measures.

Information is available from researchers who specialize in measuring the quality of life in certain types of patients. One example is the Participation and Quality of Life (Par-Qol) project (http://www.parqol.com/), which has a focus on rehabilitation in patients with spinal cord injury. If you are working in a specialty area, ask colleagues about common instruments or measures that they have used.

When you search for various health-related instruments, in addition to reviewing the content in the instrument, examine the possibilities regarding administration. Many have different smartphone apps, computer-input variations, or phone-based systems for electronic patient-reported outcomes. Electronic diaries are another option for patients where symptoms can be inputted in real time and transferred.

Discover
A useful toolkit that provides online inspection of actual questions and portions of questionnaires is the PhenX Toolkit. It was designed to facilitate phenotypic research for Genome-wide Association Studies. Go to the main page (https://www.phenxtoolkit.org/) and click on QuickStart. You are not required to create an account but if you wish to do so, registration is free. Select the Search button and insert a typical patient-reported outcome, such as "pain." If you select the Protocol Toothache and Orofacial Pain, you can see the actual questions under Protocol Text. You can also see the source, the personnel and training required, equipment needs, standards, requirements, and other practical aspects of administration. The Personnel and Training Required information can be very useful when designing the study and setting up the protocol. Feel free to explore the site.

How to Select an Instrument

There are thousands of questionnaires and instruments used in human research studies so it may be difficult to choose among the instruments available. For comparative effectiveness research, there are several considerations that are important in this regard:

- **Validity.** How well does the instrument measure what it is intended to measure?
- **Reliability.** Does the instrument yield the same results when repeated?
- **Comparability.** Can this instrument be used to compare across domains and diseases?
- **Target population.** Is this instrument suitable for the population being studied?
- **Literacy.** Is the instrument available in the language desired and at the appropriate literacy level?
- **Administration.** How is this instrument going to be applied (web-based, stand-alone computer, paper, self-administered)?
- **Burden.** Does the instrument pose a significant burden to participants (time to complete, effort)?
- **Objective.** Does this instrument fit the conceptual framework and study objectives?

There are several aspects of validity. These include construct validity, content validity, and criterion validity. Construct validity relates to whether the items in the instrument are appropriate or suitable and whether they reflect the desired domains for the particular area of interest. Content validity relates to whether the items in the instrument fully represent the domains being measured. Criterion validity relates to how well the items agree with similar valid measures. In addition to validity considerations, reliability, comparability, responsiveness to detecting changes over time, and target population should be evaluated. Instruments are available for specific populations such as children, adolescents, older adults, males and females, and patients with specific conditions or diseases. Administration of the instrument is a consideration as well; some instruments are self-administered while others require interviewers. The burden placed on participants is another aspect to consider. Often the length of the instrument (number of items) must be weighed against the likelihood that all participants would complete the assessments. Of critical importance is whether the specific instrument matches the outcomes that are intended for the research study.

Life Years

There are various outcomes that measure a healthy lifespan. Healthy life years is a measure of the number of remaining years that an individual is expected to live without disability. As an alternative, disability-adjusted life years is a measure of the number of years lost due to disability. It is often used by the World Health Organization to measure the burden of disease. In effect, these measures not only capture health or disability, but incorporate the time spent in these states as well. Therefore, age when the disability first occurred has a considerable impact on these measures.

> **Take A Look**
> Search online for the "WHO world report on disability" (http://www.who.int/disabilities/world_report/2011/en/index.html). You can download the report without charge. Examine how disability was determined and how it varies over various dimensions. Look at the overall scores of capacity and performance in selected health conditions such as stroke, depression, Parkinson's disease, and others. Do the findings for migraine and low back pain versus traumatic brain injury surprise you?

Primary and Secondary Outcomes

When planning a study, it is not uncommon to select several outcomes of interest. In fact, it is often wise to include several outcomes in trials or longitudinal studies because, from the viewpoint of the patient, knowledge of both beneficial and harmful effects of a given therapy would want to be known. If I use this particular treatment, what is the range of benefits and are there any adverse effects? Some of the outcomes may be patient reported and others may relate to conventional research outcomes such as remission rates of cancer or 30-day survival. For most research studies, a primary endpoint is chosen and the sample size calculations reflect the ability to detect this primary outcome, given the therapies under investigation and the characteristics of the study participants. Secondary endpoints are also frequently selected during the study design. In comparative effectiveness research, often a wide range of outcomes is incorporated into the study design because the intent of this research is to assess occurrences in the real world.

> **Discover**
> Go to a database of clinical trials such as the International Clinical Trials Registry Platform of the World Health Organization (http://apps.who.int/trialsearch/) or Clinicaltrials.gov. Search for any topic of interest to you and look at several trials. What types of primary outcomes did the investigators use? What are the secondary outcomes?

Dimensions of the Outcome

A critical aspect of research design is the evaluation of how the outcome is to be measured. Technically, this involves specific issues regarding the type of instrument used for measurement, and the metrics associated with this outcome. At the conclusion of a study, the results are quantified and statistics are often used to explain the differences between what occurred after one type of therapy versus the other. Epidemiologic measures are important to understand, because they represent common ways in which health outcomes are explained and evaluated in health-related research. They provide meaning to health-related occurrences in patients and populations. If you are new to this area, below are a few examples of simple health measures:

- **Percentages or proportions.** These measures are perhaps the most frequent and may be used to measure the prevalence of an event. For this metric, the people in the numerator are a subset of the people in the denominator. Listed are some examples used in health care:
  - 30-day mortality is the proportion (or percentage) of people who died within 30 days from the start of observation. This can be 30 days from the start of the study intervention, or 30 days from any specified occurrence in a specified group of people.
  - Case fatality is the proportion (or percentage) of people who died among those with a particular condition or disease. 10% case fatality would indicate that, of those people who had the disease, 10% died. In this measure, the time is not explicitly incorporated although, if this information were available, it would be helpful to report.

- **Rates.** Rates include information regarding time in the denominator, as well as information regarding the number of people affected. Rates are often expressed as the number of people with an event in the numerator, and the person–time at risk in the denominator. Listed are some examples used in health care.
  - **Rates of disease incidence.** Cancer incidence rates are given by the Surveillance Epidemiology and End Results (SEER) program in the United States (http://seer.cancer.gov/). These refer to the new (or incident) cases of cancer that have occurred over time. Using data from 2006 to 2010, the incidence of lung cancer in men was 74.3/100,000 person-years, and the incidence in women was 51.9/100,000 person-years (or alternately, 51.9 cases per 100,000 persons per year). If you go to the SEER site, you can see the incidence rates as well as the mortality rates for different types of cancer.
  - **Mortality rates.** These can be for an entire population or for specific segments of a population such as infant mortality rate or child mortality rate. Infant mortality rates are expressed as number of deaths per 1,000 live births.

Explore
Check out the visual representation of case fatality for different diseases at this site: http://www.informationisbeautiful.net/2009/fatal-infection/.

¤ **Means and medians.** For some outcomes reported on continuous scales, the arithmetic mean can be used. In clinical situations where there are may be outliers, median values may be used. An example would be the median length of stay in the hospital, which tends to be right skewed.

> **Take A Look**
> Rankings of countries throughout the world by rates of infant mortality are freely available (http://en.wikipedia.org/wiki/List_of_countries_by_infant_mortality_rate). Take a look at the variation in this measure worldwide.

Probabilities and odds are commonly used in comparative effectiveness research. Probability is one of most basic ways to express frequency. Within 100 people, the event occurs in 20 people. The probability of this event is 0.2. This is often expressed as a percentage (20%). Odds are another basic measure. Within 100 people, the event occurs in 20 people and does not occur in the remaining 80 people. The odds of the event occurring are 0.25 to 1 (or 20/80). The odds of the event not occurring are 4 to 1 (or 80/20).

Use the preposition "in" for probabilities, as in "There is a 1 in 5 probability that the event will occur." In probability, the people in the numerator are also in the denominator. The numerator is a subset of the denominator. Use the preposition "to" for odds. Odds are just a ratio of two numbers. The people in the numerator are *not* in the denominator. These are different people. The odds of the event not occurring are 4 to one. Four people do not experience the event while one person does. This agrees with the 1 in 5 probability whereby out of five people, one person experienced the event. Knowledge of these basic frequencies is important for clinical researchers, since such measures are used frequently in the medical literature as well as with the general public. It is not uncommon to see probabilities and odds expressed incorrectly in the general media, so your knowledge of the correct measures will help everyone to understand these better.

Comparative effectiveness research involves comparison and there are several general ways to contrast outcomes in groups. One is to calculate a ratio of two measures (divide one measure by the other), and another is to calculate the difference between two measures (subtract one measure from the other). Both such measures can be considered "estimates of effect" in that, when the frequency of the outcome in those who received therapy A is compared to the frequency of the outcome with therapy B, this gives one an impression or estimate of the comparative effects of the therapies.

Common measures to compare two therapies in the context of comparative effectiveness research are risk ratio (risk of the outcome in one group divided by the outcome risk in the comparator group), rate ratio (outcome rate in the intervention group divided by outcome rate in the comparator), and odds ratio (odds of the outcome in one group versus the odds of the outcome in the other). Sometimes the term "relative risk" is used, and can indicate either a risk ratio or a rate ratio. All of these measures range from zero to infinity. If you think about these measures, it becomes clear that when the frequency of the outcome is the same in both groups, the risk ratio would be one. This would occur under the null hypothesis —that is, there is no difference in outcomes between the two therapies. If, however, the risk ratio were 2.0, we would say that the risk of the outcome is twice as great in patients receiving therapy A as in patients receiving therapy B. If, however, the risk ratio were 0.75, we would say that the risk of the outcome in patients receiving therapy A is less than, or 0.75 times, that of patients receiving therapy B. Another way to say this would be that patients receiving therapy A have a 25% reduction in risk as patients receiving therapy B (just subtract from 0.75 from the null).

Many researchers are accustomed to seeing relative risks where the reference category consists of people not receiving a treatment (a control group without treatment or a placebo group). Interpretations of relative risks deserve special attention in comparative effectiveness research because the reference category (denominator for a relative risk) refers to a different type of therapy. There is no placebo group. This is because the definition of comparative effectiveness research is the comparison of two or more types of potentially useful interventions or therapies. As a researcher and reader of the medical literature, pay attention to which group of people is placed in the denominator. That is, if you see a relative risk of 2.0, you have to ask yourself first whether therapy A yields twice the risk of therapy B, or whether therapy B yields twice the risk of therapy A. This should be evident from the description of the methods in the research study.

If the final estimate of effect in a comparative effectiveness research study is an absolute risk difference, one also must be a bit careful when describing differences. Here we technically mean mathematical differences—subtracting one frequency from another. In the medical literature and the general media, the word "difference" is sometimes casually used. It is possible to see relative risks at the end of a study where the authors also refer to differences in outcomes for the various treatment groups (even though the comparison involves division and not subtraction). This is just an idiosyncratic aspect of the English language. Technically, the word difference can be used to describe general contrasts between groups. Other times, difference refers specifically to mathematical subtraction.

If you are conducting a trial or a longitudinal study, you might consider reporting both relative risks and risk differences. Sometimes such measures can tell slightly different stories. For rare conditions you can sometimes obtain large relative risks, but the risk difference can be quite modest. For conditions that are common, sometimes the relative risk is not dramatic but the risk difference can be quite large. For example, suppose you wish to improve activities of daily living in a particular group of patients with mild disability. The overall ability to prepare a meal independently is, say, 70%. The outcome is fairly common overall, so one would not expect huge relative risks at the end of this study. But you may end up with 20% more of the patients being able to make meals independently after a certain intervention compared to another. This 20% risk difference may translate, in a large population, to a significant number of people who are capable of doing something that is incredibly important to independent living. However, the relative risk (0.9/0.7=1.29) looks quite modest. In general, risk differences speak more to the expected volume of effect. This can have important implications for health policy.

In another example, let's suppose that a researcher wants to assess the effectiveness of a specific stem cell therapy for the treatment of a specific type of cancer. The two treatment groups are (1) stem cell therapy plus high-dose chemotherapy, versus (2) high-dose chemotherapy alone. When chemotherapy only is administered, the five-year survival rate is 4%. When the combined therapy is administered, the survival rate is 12%. The relative risk is 3.0 (12%/4%). Within the medical literature, a relative risk of 3.0 (with a tight confidence interval) is generally considered a strong indicator of effectiveness of one therapy versus another. The risk difference, however, is 8%, which looks rather modest. From this evidence the new therapy appears promising, but still, the survival rate for patients remains low for both therapies.

Regardless of the variety of approaches seen in the medical literature for describing the outcome results, there are a few concepts that are routinely utilized in comparative effectiveness research that you may already know. These two concepts are as follows:

- **Confidence interval.** Confidence intervals are a way of assessing the variability in your findings. In effect, they enable you to make statements regarding the wider reference population from the study data. Suppose that in a trial we find that 10% of the patients died after receiving therapy A, and 14% of patients died after receiving therapy B. We could just report these measures and say that there was a 4% difference in mortality rates. Does this mean that 10% of all such patients will die after receiving therapy A and 14% of all such patients will die after receiving therapy B? We cannot make this statement, because, frankly, we do not really know exactly what would happen in other people. But we could make a pretty good guess at what would happen in other people if we used a confidence interval. A confidence interval is a way of going from our particular sample (study) to the larger reference population. Confidence intervals of 95% are widely used. So if we, as researchers, calculate the 95% confidence interval around the 4% difference that we found in our study, we might end up with 95% CI = 3.1% to 5.2%. The 95% confidence interval straddles the 4% difference. The confidence interval always goes around the estimate of effect—which is 4% in this study. The lower limit (3.1%)

goes below it and the upper limit goes above it (5.2%). What then does the 95% confidence interval actually mean in terms of the reference population? It means this: *If a researcher were to take 100 random samples from the reference population, then in 95 of these samples, the difference in mortality rates would fall between 3.1% and 5.2%.* So we are pretty confident that the true difference in mortality—in all such patients—is between 3.1% and 5.2%. This is a way of extrapolating from our study to expectations in all such patients.

¤ **P-value.** The *P*-value is another mechanism by which we can use our study results to say something about the reference population in general. Using the same example of a 4% difference in mortality rates between patients receiving therapy A versus therapy B, we might calculate a *P*-value of 0.002 for this difference. The "p" in *P*-value stands for probability. *The P-value is the probability of attaining our study results or more extreme study results if, in the reference population, therapy A has the same death rate as therapy B.* So a *P*-value of 0.002 indicates that the probability of finding the 4% difference in mortality rates (10% with therapy A and 14% with therapy B) or more extreme results (that is, more than 4% difference) would occur two times in 1000, if the mortality rates were actually equal in the reference population. This is a small probability, and it indicates that we are not likely to find these study results just by chance alone. If the results are not likely due to chance (also called random error), then what is the likely cause? If we had a well-designed trial, it's likely due to therapy A actually being better than therapy B in preventing death. That's why this *P*-value is important. *It is one way in which we can guess, from existing information, what is likely to occur in the future.* If I were a patient with this condition and had a choice between therapy A versus B, I'd certainly choose therapy A, all else being equal. We already demonstrated that this finding was not likely due to chance.

Both confidence intervals and *P*-values are indices that assist us from going from study results to making predictions in other people. These indices are used in inferential statistics; we are making inferences from our study results to the reference population. There are other types of procedures used in data analyses that can be utilized in explaining the study results as well. One such general procedure is to use a Bayesian approach. With Bayesian inference, the researcher uses prior information regarding the probability of an event and combines it with additional information to assess the probability of the event. That is, both prior data and new data from a particular study are utilized to assess the post-probability of occurrence. It is a valid approach as well; it's just a different way of looking at the world.

At the end of a comparative effectiveness research study, there is another measure that may be useful. This measure is called the Number Needed to Treat (NNT). Mathematically, the number needed to treat is just the inverse of the absolute difference. It is 1 divided by the outcome risk in those patients receiving therapy A minus the outcome risk in those patients receiving therapy B. In common language, it is the number of patients needed to receive therapy A in order for one additional patient to benefit (above that of the comparison treatment B). If therapy A improves functioning in 40% of patients and therapy B improves functioning in 30% of patients, then the risk difference is 10%. The inverse of this is 10 (1/0.1). In terms of this example, 10 people would need to be treated with therapy A instead of therapy B in order for one additional person to improve their functioning. A low number needed to treat indicates a more effective therapy. A high number needed to treat indicates a less effective therapy.

Check It Out

There are central sites whereby the Number Needed to Treat (and the Number Needed to Harm) are listed for various therapies that have been evaluated through randomized controlled trials. One such site is TheNNT.com (http://www.thennt.com/). Search for it and browse through the reviews. It is an easy way to find information regarding effective and ineffective therapies. You can also scan the relative effectiveness of various therapies by looking at the NNT on the Bandolier site (http://www.medicine.ox.ac.uk/bandolier/band50/b50-8.html). Which treatments tend to be quite effective (with a low NNT)?

5

The Design

Design is of the utmost importance. Design dictates the information to be collected and provides the structure by which entities can be compared. Design encompasses who will be studied, in what time frame, in what manner, the services to be compared, and the outcomes chosen. The design of a study not only provides the backbone, but the organizational elements attached to this backbone.

The Scientific Method

Science involves two basic processes. One is experimentation. The other is observation. A hypothesis is formed. Through either observation or experimentation, data are collected regarding the factors involved and conclusions are reached based on the findings. Elements of the scientific method are frequently found in ordinary life. Observation is necessary for survival. It is not an accident that humans have evolved with keen senses in which to observe the world. Seeing, hearing, tasting, touching, and smelling the environment around us has a direct impact on our day-to-day functioning and overall health. It is natural that observation would form an important aspect of evidence. We frequently practice elements of experimentation in our daily lives as well through trial and error. Both experimentation and observation form the foundation of evidence-based discovery and have considerable consequences on the decisions we make and the outcomes we experience.

WHAT IS A TRIAL?

A trial is when an investigator purposefully changes or intervenes in the ordinary course of life to see what occurs afterwards. Sometimes trials are called interventional studies or experiments. Human trials tend to be a bit different from experiments conducted in some of the basic sciences. In basic science trials, the researcher often tries to make everything as similar as possible across all experimental groups except for the treatment under investigation. Then, when you notice a difference in the results between the treatment and the control, it probably is due to the treatment itself. That is, many of the extraneous factors are controlled and therefore the treatment effect (if it does occur) can be more noticeable. Trials in humans are not as constrained. In human trials, the social, cultural, and physical environment cannot be totally identical for each person in the study. Our homes, our families, our networks are different. What one person may be exposed to could be quite different from another.

Some elements of trial design are evident in ordinary life. Have you ever seen a group of children who, after school, play a quick game of football or softball? Two captains are chosen. A coin is tossed to see which captain goes first. Based on the results of the toss, one of the captains chooses a classmate to be a player on his or her team. Then the other captain chooses a player. The captains go back and forth, selecting players until everyone is chosen. The ballgame proceeds. At the end, the team with the highest score wins. It is a comparison of abilities—one team versus the other. It is a trial of two teams in which an outcome is reached. A factor making this trial somewhat of a balanced competition is that the players are chosen one at a time for either team, with those having better athletic abilities generally chosen first. This, in effect, is a type of design. This design includes very simple randomization (by a single coin toss) that is intended to match the teams somewhat in expected abilities before the start of the game. And the design is so simple that children do it naturally.

A trial is essentially any intervention, the occurrence of which is provoked by research investigators. A trial can be a test of a screening procedure or medication use or invasive surgery, all with the intent to observe outcomes after the therapies. It could be a change in practice or a change in diet in order to see the effects. It may be an alteration in methods of delivery for certain routine services, with a measurement of patient outcomes afterwards.

WHAT IS DESIGN?

The design of a comparative effectiveness research study includes the essential components of the research question and incorporates the necessary elements to answer the question. It includes a detailed structure of the study type and the features of the study (e.g., randomization, parallel arms), defines the procedures for analyses, and outlines the protocol for implementation. Design includes the following elements:

- ¤ A statement of the research question(s) or scientific hypotheses.
- ¤ A description of the sample and the reference population, including the number of subjects to be enrolled or investigated.
- ¤ The source of the sample including locations and calendar time of the study period.

- A description of all active comparators to be investigated.
- A description of the outcomes including primary and secondary endpoints.
- A design structure in context, with a statement of study type and the specifications of design features within the study. Often this includes a diagrammatic model.
- An outline for data management and a description of the data analyses.

This process begins with formulating the overall objective of the study, but may include several specific aims. The planning process involves a careful examination of the options available and a consideration of the factors necessary to provide sufficient evidence in order to answer the question(s) of interest. A visual representation of the design structure is advised, as well as the written description.

The design of a study is not its analysis. Study design is not a regression equation or an analytic procedure. The study design explains who, what, where, when, and how. The design is the set-up and, ultimately, design trumps analysis.

> **RULE OF THUMB**: Design trumps analysis.

A poor design can rarely be overcome by analyses. In order to answer a specific research question one must have the appropriate sample from the reference population (or the entire population) taken at the appropriate time, with the comparators and outcomes of interest, and using a suitable design structure. The design should fit the research question.

Let's start with a fine design: the randomized controlled trial. For purposes of comparative effectiveness research, this design is slightly renamed as a randomized trial with active comparators.

Randomized Trial with Active Comparators

Historically, the types of studies that best typify clinical research are randomized controlled trials, denoted as RCT in the medical literature. Such trials involve randomization of patients to treatment groups and include a control or a comparison group. There are various options regarding the type and timing of the randomization process, as well as options regarding how and when the comparator groups are involved. There are also several choices regarding the outcome measurements and the analyses. For purposes of comparative effectiveness research, randomized trials are planned with an active comparator in each study group.

The basic structure of a trial is prospective—from subject enrollment, assignment to treatments, and follow-up to determine the outcomes. Sometimes

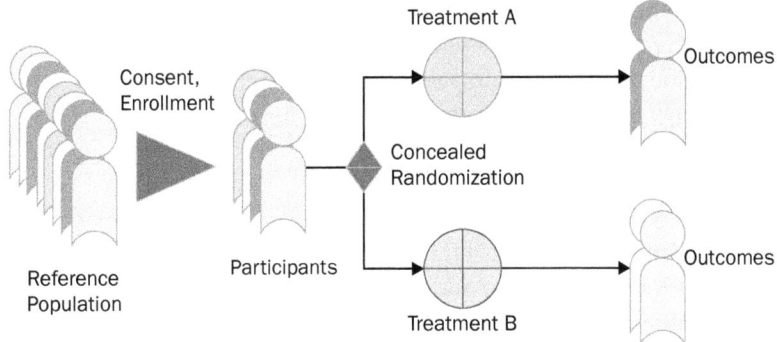

FIGURE 5.1 Randomized Trial with Two Comparators.

one sees the phrase "prospective trial" written, but every trial is prospective in nature (the exception may be a natural experiment). An example of a randomized trial with two comparators is given in Figure 5.1.

Listed below are some conventional elements of trial design:

- **Arms.** An arm in a trial refers to the group of people who receive one of the comparators. If therapy A is being compared to procedure B, then the subjects in the therapy A group form one arm and the subjects receiving procedure B form the other arm. Many trials have two arms, although a trial may have more than two arms (representing more than two comparators). In comparative effectiveness research, all arms are most often active comparator arms. That is, at the beginning of the study, the therapy in each arm is considered a potentially effective treatment to be tested.
- **Controlled.** A controlled trial is a trial with an arm receiving an alternative therapy for purposes of comparison. Historically, the control would be a group that received a placebo or no treatment in a randomized controlled trial. However, in comparative effectiveness research, this control or comparator should be explicitly described and should constitute a suitable viable therapeutic alternative for an individual or population.
- **Parallel.** A parallel trial is one in which the comparator arms are administered during the same calendar time period.
- **Run-in period.** One feature that has been incorporated into some randomized controlled trials is a run-in period. This is a short period of time prior to randomization when potential subjects can be screened for compliance and baseline characteristics prior to study entrance. The run-in period can be considered a short test period prior to the start of the trial when the investigator ensures that all subjects are ready for entrance. A run-in period prior to

randomization has been used to ensure that subjects meet eligibility requirements so that baseline measurements can be made. In some previous studies, certain patients who did not tolerate the drug or therapy were excluded prior to the trial. Since one of the purposes of comparative effectiveness research is to discover which types of patients will respond to therapies during usual clinical practice, any exclusions should be judicious before considering this option.

- **Blinding.** Blinding (also called masking) is a particular design feature in which information is purposefully withheld to reduce potential bias. If the researchers suspect that knowledge of treatment assignment may alter patients' responses or influence the way in which clinicians record the outcome or interact with the subjects, it may be useful to consider the incorporation of blinding into the design. Sometimes patients or their providers may have preconceived notions regarding the effects of the therapies, which may influence the outcome. This could introduce unnecessary bias into the study. In a typical randomized controlled trial, the participants may not be told whether they are receiving drug A or drug B. When subjects are blinded to which treatment arm they are receiving, this is called a single-blind trial. When both the subjects and the investigators are blinded to which treatment each subject is receiving, this is called a double-blind trial.

Consider

Suppose that there is a team of 14 investigators who are collaborating on a large trial. They all participate in the design. A few conduct the randomization, some are involved with patient enrollment, others administer the therapies to the participants, and others assist with arranging the follow-up phone calls. Several investigators assess the primary and secondary outcomes during clinic visits. Other colleagues assist with data entry, programming, and statistical analyses. If blinding were possible, which of these investigators would be the most likely candidates for blinding so as to reduce the likelihood of selection bias (errors in how subjects are selected for the study or assigned to each of the arms) or information bias (measurement error related to the therapies or the outcomes)?

Blinding is more commonly used when the comparators are two drugs, whereby the pharmacist can design similar-looking drugs. As you might imagine, blinding cannot often be utilized when comparing two different types of therapies. If one of the therapies involves a procedure and the other involves the use of a biologic, the researcher may not be able to conceal such differences. In comparative effectiveness research, the use of placebos or sham procedures are not usually tested because the comparators should reflect options that would be considered during ordinary life. Such trials in which both the participants and the researchers know the group assignment are sometimes called open randomized trials or open label trials.

Blinding is not just a design feature relegated to randomized trials. It should be utilized when possible for nonrandomized studies as well. Consider a trial in which the outcome is microbiologically confirmed bloodstream infection. The outcome is generated by the individuals working in the pathology laboratory who process and read the results from the blood cultures. There may be no need for these individuals to know the assignment groups in the study. In this instance, you could include blinding of the treatment assignment to those individuals who ascertain the outcome. When publishing your results, you could then indicate that the laboratory technicians were blinded to treatment assignment.

Another design feature in a randomized trial is concealment of randomization:

- **Concealment.** Concealment of randomization refers to withholding knowledge regarding the specific randomization procedure in order to reduce potential selection bias. Concealment occurs before the subjects are assigned and is usually done by the statistician or analyst who conducts the randomization procedure. Then, at the time that the subjects are assigned to treatment groups, blinding can be implemented. Concealment of the randomization procedure is not the same as blinding, although if you have not yet conducted a trial, they may appear similar. Both involve withholding information, but these are two different design features. Concealment pertains to withholding information regarding the randomization procedure itself and sometimes is called allocation concealment. Blinding refers to withholding knowledge regarding the treatment assignments to participants and/or investigators during the course of the trial. Blinding may not be possible if the therapies are noticeably different such as comparisons between drug therapy and a surgical procedure. However, even if blinding cannot be implemented, allocation concealment should always be performed in a randomized trial.

For randomized trials, the investigator has several options available for studying comparisons. There are studies which provide **within-person comparisons**. That is, for a given patient, the intervention would be tested and any effects would be assessed after the intervention and during comparison periods. Examples of such trials are N-of-1 trials and crossover trials. Another option includes studies with **between-person comparisons**. That is, one intervention is given to some individuals and another intervention is given to others. The conventional randomized controlled trial is in this category, as are factorial trials with multiple arms.

A further option includes studies in which there are **cluster comparisons** (or group comparisons). In these trials, interventions are administered to clusters (or groups) of people and are compared to interventions administered to other groups of people. Clustering can also be performed in crossover trials that involve within-group comparisons, whereby interventions are given to groups of people at different time periods. Clustering works well for studies in which patients are naturally grouped, such as patients with the same primary care provider. In this instance, each primary care practitioner defines the cluster and the patients are nested within each of these clusters. We sometimes call this a two-level hierarchical design.

Randomization

HOW DOES ONE RANDOMIZE?

Randomization is a procedure in which each participant in the trial has an equal (or preset) probability of being assigned to the study groups. It is a distinctive element of trials. One of the purposes of randomization is to avoid selection bias. That is, one would not want an investigator to selectively choose certain patients to be given a treatment because of their knowledge or beliefs regarding these particular patients, their disease severity, or the particular treatments. It is not uncommon for people to have preferences for a given treatment based on their past experiences. If the patients choose their own study group or the investigator chooses it for them, these choices may lead to an unfair comparison between the study groups because of these baseline differences in the types of people within each study group. Another purpose of randomization is to minimize differences in the study groups by other factors that may be related to both the outcome and the treatment. Such third factors (associated with both the treatment and outcome) are sometimes called confounding factors or confounders. For example, sometimes the choice of a therapy depends on the patient's age, and, in addition, the outcome (e.g., regaining arm strength) may also be a function of age. In this instance, age could be a potential confounding factor. If one randomizes a large number of subjects, the age distribution in the study groups will tend to equalize. However, randomization of smaller groups of people can, by chance, result in unequal distributions of various study characteristics such as age. As the number of people randomized increases, the likelihood of differences in potential confounders decreases.

Definition
Within the context of comparative effectiveness research, a confounder is an entity that is related to the comparators as well as to the outcome, but is not a consequence of any of the comparators (i.e., not within the causal pathway from comparator to outcome).

That being said, in a randomized controlled trial with concurrent parallel arms, the investigator will never have equally matched patient characteristics by assigning people to two or more mutually exclusive groups. This is because there are always complex genetic differences among people that are not exactly the same in the study groups. Everyone on the earth is unique. Besides the genetic differences, think about the unique combination of different disorders and injuries that an individual can experience over time, and combine this with their treatment therapies for these disorders and the degree to which they adhered to these treatments. These things happen differently in people. Even identical twins, who share their genetic makeup, experience some differences in their environment throughout their lifetimes and may exhibit epigenetic variation. The closest equalization of potential confounding factors might be the randomization of identical twins raised in the same environment. While randomization of different people to different groups is often hailed in the medical literature as being the true test of whether a given intervention works or does not work, such studies can provide very good evidence—but they are not perfect.

Randomization, nevertheless, is a strong design feature and is important to include if ethical and feasible. Sometimes investigators may be reticent regarding whether individuals would be willing to be randomized to receive certain therapies. But conduct a quick search of the medical literature on the comparators or similar comparators of interest. You might find that other researchers have found creative ways to administer an intervention and to incorporate randomization. For example, it would be unethical to randomize individuals to known carcinogens—say, conventional cigarettes versus smokeless cigarettes. But it may be possible to randomize individuals to smoking cessation strategies for both such cigarette users. It is not the same hypothesis to be tested, but it may be similar enough to be of interest.

Considerations prior to randomization. There are several common questions to be answered prior to conducting the randomization.

- At the start of the trial, are all subjects identified so that they can be randomized at the same calendar time? In this instance, the individual performing the concealed randomization procedure may assign the subjects to the treatment groups all at once.
- Will the subjects be enrolled at different times throughout the course of the trial? In this instance, the randomizer will develop the procedures necessary to assign the treatment to each patient as he or she enters the trial. This scenario is very common in clinical trials; patients are enrolled over the course of time.
- Will each subject receive only one treatment assignment in the study, or will the subjects be assigned different treatment assignments over time? If there are different treatment assignments over time for a given subject, the randomizer will prepare the necessary randomized *sequence* for each subject. This would occur in a typical crossover trial or N-of-1 trial.
- Are groups of people being randomized together as a cluster? There may be instances in which all patients from a certain practice or therapy group may be randomized as a unit. Randomization of clusters may be a common feature in some comparative effectiveness studies.

- Are other units being randomized rather than an individual person? It is possible to randomize other entities, such as body parts that have bilateral symmetry. For example, the right and left knees of the same person may be randomized to different treatments.

Each of the above scenarios may alter the randomization procedure. There is no universal randomization procedure used in every trial, other than the general requirement of some mechanism for generating random numbers with the assignment based on a specific probability. Most often, the results yield an equal probability of being assigned to one of two study arms. The randomization procedures chosen reflect elements of the study design that are specific to the underlying scientific hypothesis. It is important for the investigator conducting the randomization to consult with the principal investigator and coinvestigators regarding the elements of the design in order to tailor the randomization to the particular study.

For vast majority of randomized controlled trials, *the underlying principle of randomization is that each person has an equal (or preset) probability of being assigned to the study arms.* For some trials, the investigators may purposefully want an unequal number of subjects in the study arms. In this instance, the underlying principle is that each person has the predetermined specific probability of being assigned to each of the treatment groups.

How to conduct simple randomization. When conducting this procedure, the investigator must keep in mind the general underlying principle—that each person should have an equal (or preset) probability of being assigned to each study arm.

- First, identify your source of random numbers. There are several sources: (1) computer generated random numbers, (2) sources of true random numbers, and (3) printed tables of random numbers. Computer random number generators usually employ a mathematical algorithm, and technically, are pseudorandom number generators. These are often available in common statistical programs. Although they are not true random numbers, such computer generators are used extensively within medical studies. Truly random numbers generated from atmospheric noise (http://www.random.org) are also available. Various printed tables of random numbers have been historically available in statistical textbooks, but have essentially been replaced by computer generation.
- Randomization involves a procedure whereby some rules must be initially specified. Let's walk through a simple example in which you expect to enroll 400 patients to two study arms (200 in each arm). In one arm, the patients will receive behavioral therapy. In the other arm, the patients will receive incentives. The patients will be enrolled in a clinic over an eight-month time period. We can generate a random set of numbers with apportionment to two groups. First, we create

unique study identification numbers for each of the 400 perspective participants within our computer file. Second, we decide that behavioral therapy will be assigned to group 0 and the incentive arm will be assigned to group 1 (each group will have an equal probability of selection so that either one could have been given the "0" or the "1" – but we must decide this first). We go back to our computer file and generate a random number and apportion it to two groups (0 and 1). Now we have a file with each person's identification number (our first variable), and we also have another variable indicating their study assignment, which was generated through randomization. For each study, the exact step-by-step procedures may vary somewhat, depending upon the study design and which computer program that you use for randomization. There are straightforward procedures to utilize in the major statistical packages. For each computer program, be careful to read the instructions beforehand so that the procedure is conducted correctly. Apportionment can be done for two, three, four, or more study arms.

The above process is an example of simple randomization, but if an investigator conducts simple randomization without any other procedures, one problem that can occur (by chance) is an unequal number of subjects assigned to each arm. Suppose that in the study with 400 prospective patients, the investigators could only enroll 350 patients in the study. Not every patient wanted to be randomized and participate in the study. With 350 total subjects, there could be—just by chance—180 assigned to behavioral therapy and 170 assigned to incentives. There are a few methods to ensure that an equal number of people will be in each group. The most common approach is called blocking.

- **Blocking** is a procedure used to equalize the number of subjects within each treatment group when performing randomization. This is particularly important for trials in which people are recruited over time. If simple randomization is conducted and there is an imbalance in the number of patients assigned to the study arms at a given time, this could be problematic in several ways. There could be temporal changes that cannot be controlled (e.g., seasonal differences) that could possibly influence exposures over time. There could also be an instance in which interim effects of treatment are assessed (as planned beforehand) and, in these situations, it may be important to have equal sample sizes in each arm. This tends to enhance statistical power (i.e., the ability to find a difference if there really is one). If you conduct randomization with blocking, it is relatively straightforward. In a simple example, first set a block size. Let's say that we choose a block size of 8 in which patients are randomized to two study arms (A and B) over a period of time. We want to ensure that, within every group of 8 patients, 4 would be assigned to A and 4 would be assigned to B. Examples of some of the possible permutations for study assignment are ABABABAB, AABBAABB, ABBAABBA, ABBBAAAB, and so forth. The entire set of possible permutations is first delineated, and then such blocks are randomly chosen. As the first 8 patients are given their random assignments, it is ensured that within these first 8 patients, 4 people will be assigned to study arm A and 4 will be assigned to study arm B. For the next 8 patients, 4 will be assigned to A and 4 to B. This continues throughout the trial. These are sometimes called **random permuted blocks**.

Determining Block Size. After the decision is made to use blocking, the investigator has a choice regarding the size of the blocks. Below are some considerations.

- Small block sizes are often discouraged because it is more likely that someone could guess the order of assignment based on the treatment group of the previous patients. If the block size is 2 and the first patient receives treatment A, then one knows that the second patient will receive treatment B.
- The block size should be a multiple of the number of treatment groups. If there are three treatment groups, one could use a block size of 6, 9, 12, 15, 18, and so on. If one used a block size of 5 with three treatment groups, then it would not be possible for an equal number of people assigned to each of the three treatments within a given block.
- To decrease predictability, it is useful to randomize the block size. That is, it is often wise to conduct one extra design feature—randomize *block sizes* first. So, instead of just using one fixed block size, choose several block sizes (let's say we choose block sizes from 4 to 12). In a trial with two treatment groups, the block sizes must be an even number because people are assigned to two groups. Then you randomly generate a series of blocks of these sizes (e.g., block sizes 12, 4, 6, 10, 8, 6, 8, etc.; note that this is sampling with replacement since each block size can be used more than once), and subjects are assigned to the study arms equally within each block. Since it is important to conceal the randomization process from the investigators who are enrolling patients, changing the size of the blocks makes it more difficult to predict the group to which the next patient will be assigned. In this instance, blocked randomization was used with random block size and an equal allocation ratio (which just means the same number in each arm). Do not confuse "random permuted blocks" with "random block size." Random permuted blocks just refers to blocked randomization. *Random block size* refers to an additional design feature in which the size of the block was chosen randomly.

If you conduct this extra step, you can then write in the methods section of your paper that "random permuted blocks were generated for treatment assignment, with random block sizes of 4, 6, 8, 10, and 12." If you do not randomly choose block size, you can report that "random permuted blocks were generated for treatment assignment with a block size of 8."

STRATIFIED RANDOM SAMPLING

There are other elements that can be built into the randomization procedure as well. One such design factor is called **stratified randomization**. Stratified randomization is a procedure that is conducted to minimize the differences in the study arms based on patient characteristics that are known at the start of the trial. For example, some trials are stratified by disease severity at the onset to ensure that study groups are balanced by this characteristic. If response to therapies is associated with disease severity and the outcome is also associated with disease severity, we call this potential confounding because disease severity may potentially confound or affect the relationship between therapy and outcome. Therefore, we would like to ensure—from the start—that there is a balance in disease severity across the study arms. We purposefully ensure that each study arm has the same proportion of people with severe disease. To conduct stratification, first decide the variable or variables for stratification. For a variable such as disease severity, you and your team of investigators would have to determine what criteria constitute more severe disease from less severe disease. Based on the total number of patients randomized to each arm, you must consider whether dividing severity into two groups is best or whether three categories of severity are better (and so forth). Let's suppose we chose two categories for severity (less severe versus more severe). Stratification is straightforward. You take the patients with less severe disease and randomize them separately to each of the study arms. Then you take the patients with more severe disease and randomize them separately to each of the study arms. It's basically just splitting the patients into the two groups (strata) and then conducting randomization (as you would normally from the examples above) within each group. Randomization occurs within the strata.

There are other randomization procedures available in addition to blocking and

> **Question** Stratified randomization seems somewhat like blocking. Are these really different?
>
> **Answer** These two procedures are actually different. Stratification is conducted to balance the study groups across various patient-relevant or baseline characteristics. Blocking is conducted to balance the study groups in terms of the number of patients in each study arm. Blocking does not ensure equalization of subjects across the treatment groups by baseline patient characteristics (that's what stratification does). Stratification does not ensure equal numbers of subjects in each arm (that's what blocking does). Many trials use both blocking and stratification when conducting randomization.

> **Discover**
> There are several online sites where you can practice randomization. Try the Research Randomizer (http://www.randomizer.org/). Put in a few numbers, as if you were designing a trial. There are many commercial randomization sites as well. Random.org provides some free services which are fun to explore.

stratification. One such technique is minimization, which strives to minimize the imbalance in baseline patient characteristics by calculating the imbalance in characteristics and using this to assign treatment group. Always check the performance of such procedures and their advantages versus disadvantages for your particular study before implementation.

Categorizing Trials: Pragmatic Versus Explanatory

Comparative effectiveness research is an effort to evaluate the effects of various therapies in real-world settings. Such randomized trials are labeled **pragmatic trials**. That is, they are trials that assess the relative benefits and risks of several therapies for a given condition under usual conditions or during routine clinical practice. This is in contrast to an **explanatory trial**, such as a double-blind randomized controlled trial of a new drug versus placebo, in which efficacy under ideal conditions is evaluated.

In pragmatic randomized trials, the eligibility criteria are broad. The study participants should reflect the types of individuals who would normally receive such therapies or services. In pragmatic trials, the delivery of the therapies (be they drugs, biologics, use of a device, communication strategies, etc.) should be feasible during usual practice for the physicians, nurse practitioners, dentists, or whoever normally delivers such services. There would be an attempt to enter a wide range of people into the trial, even if they may have different types of comorbidities or underlying differences. The study participants should reflect the types of people who would be likely to receive such therapies in usual practice. The outcomes would be meaningful to patients; that is, patient-reported outcomes would be considered. In addition, all relevant outcomes for the particular therapies under investigation would be evaluated (Tunis, 2003).

> **Discover**
> There have been guidelines and tools developed to help researchers who wish to design pragmatic trials. One such tool is called PRECIS or Pragmatic-Explanatory Continuum Indicator Summary (Thorpe, 2009). Find this online (http://www.cmaj.ca/content/180/10/E47.full.pdf). Look at the PRECIS diagrammatic wheel, which was intended to assist the design process, and read through a few examples.

In practice, there may be instances in which a team of researchers designs a randomized trial which has some elements of explanatory trials (e.g., rigid treatment protocols, exact follow-up procedures) and yet has some elements of pragmatic trials (e.g., more inclusive patient recruitment with patient-centered outcomes). There can be some overlap. This sometimes is referred to as adaptation. Frankly, categorization is of less importance than the development of abilities to take important health questions that may impact patients' lives and to build mechanisms in which to answer these questions.

Adaptive Trials

One of the more recent developments in trial design has been the willingness to incorporate changes within the structure of trials. Adaptive trials are randomized trials that allow some components of change during implementation. Based on predefined specifications at the start of the trial, changes may be allowed during the trial based on interim results. These trials can involve design elements such as adaptive randomization, adaptive arm dropping, and early stopping (based on futility or early success). For example, if one of the arms shows a higher probability of benefit, additional patients can be added to this arm. If an additional therapy becomes available (e.g., new on the market), an additional arm can be included. If it becomes clear that one treatment provides better benefit than another, the arm with the lower benefit can be dropped. If it is apparent that a specific patient subgroup experiences better outcomes after receiving a certain therapy, additional patients within this subgroup may be enrolled. Such trials, because of their iterative revisions, can sometimes achieve results faster, in a smaller number of participants, and yet yield a greater proportion of patients who received beneficial therapy. Utilization of this approach is less akin to the historical efficacy trial with a specific start and stop date, and is more akin to an evolutionary trial with continuous monitoring, refinement, and integration of novel therapies as they become available. Because adaptive trials are more closely tied to real-world conditions, they show promise for comparative effectiveness research.

Features of adaptive design that are sometimes considered are:

- **Adaptation of eligibility criteria.** After a trial begins, it may become apparent that only certain types of patients choose to participate. The baseline characteristics of patients who are enrolled do not match the types of patients who originally were expected to participate. It may be useful to reconsider the eligibility criteria and focus recruitment on the types of patients who are likely to enroll. There may be other reasons for adaption as well. For example, low recruitment numbers may indicate a need to assess the eligibility criteria to widen potential participation.
- **Adaptation due to unexpected outcomes.** When evaluating new therapies, sometimes adverse effects are seen that were not anticipated at the start of the trial. This could be due to a number of factors, such as specific dosages received by certain participants or patient characteristics that unexpectedly influence outcomes. Considerations

may be made regarding discontinuation of a certain dosage or restriction of therapy to specific types of patients.
- **Adaptation based on interim analyses showing lack of effect.** There are studies in which the treatment is administered to different groups of patients over time (e.g., group sequential designs). Sometimes it is clear when interim analyses are conducted that, even if the remaining elements of the trial were completed, there would be no difference in treatment effect in the various study arms. In such instances, it may be prudent to discontinue the trial.
- **Adaptation based on interim analyses showing beneficial effect.** On the other hand, if one of the therapies is found to be greatly more effective than anticipated in comparison to other treatments, this may also warrant consideration of early stopping and offering the therapy to all patients who may benefit.
- **Adaptation of randomization.** Occasionally, the randomization procedure may be adjusted. For example, randomized trials often use an equal allocation ratio during randomization. If, however, there is evidence of one therapy showing greater benefit than another, consideration of changing this allocation ratio may occur so that more patients are randomized to the potentially beneficial arm.
- **Adaptation of study population.** It is possible that during the course of the trial, it becomes evident that patients with a certain genetic profile or specific characteristics respond differently to the therapeutic options than at first anticipated. This information can be used to alter the study population so to target the therapies to those participants that would most likely see an effect.

Historically, adaptive trial designs have been used for specific applications. One application is called the sequential randomized controlled trial. This is often contrasted with the fixed-size randomized controlled trial.

- **Fixed-size randomized trial.** A fixed size trial is one in which the researcher determines the total number of subjects to be enrolled before starting the trial. This is done by calculating the number of subjects necessary to detect a specific treatment effect when comparing various therapies. One generally relies on data from pilot or preliminary trials, or from data or results from other studies, to estimate the probable rates of the outcome in the study arms. The ability to detect this effect is called statistical power. We often set power at either 80% or 90% before the start of a study. That is, we want to make sure that we are able to detect a specific difference in outcomes between the study arms with a certain level of confidence. For a typical trial, 80% power means that there would be an 80%

probability of rejecting the null hypothesis (of no difference in outcome rates in the treatment arms) when the null hypothesis is not true.

¤ **Sequential randomized trial.** A researcher planning a sequential trial, on the other hand, does not set a fixed sample size before the study starts. The sequential trial begins with subject recruitment and continues until one therapy proves more beneficial than the other. If no difference in benefit is evident for a given length of time, the trial is concluded showing no benefit of one therapy versus another. The time limit for determination of no benefit is preset and determined before the start of the trial. The sequential trial tends to be preferable when one therapy is expected to show clear benefits earlier than another. If it does, then the trial could conclude earlier with fewer subjects enrolled. And, if it does take a shorter amount of time to show the benefit, then the beneficial therapy could be offered to patients sooner.

One of the more common applications of adaptive trial design is called a sequential multiple assignment randomized trial or SMART (Lei, 2012). Such SMART designs have been used in the mental health field and involve multiple stages corresponding to critical decision points. At each stage, randomization is conducted and treatment options may change, based on the status of the patient during the course of the trial. In a SMART design, the same patients are observed over time but their options may change based on their progress or response to therapies. In essence, there is randomization of treatment sequences over time for patients with consideration of their changing health status. This approach has great appeal for comparative effectiveness research.

An adaptive trial must be planned carefully prior to implementation. All adaptations that are intended should be clearly specified at the start. This includes decisions regarding timing, how many adaptations are to be determined with regard to results and participants, the types of analyses, and the primary endpoint. If adaptations are utilized, the CONSORT statement can be utilized with modifications (Consolidated Standards of Reporting Trials available at http://www.consort-statement.org/consort-statement/ or at http://www.consort-statement.org/extensions/designs/pragmatic-trials/). This statement provides guidance regarding inclusion and exclusion criteria, study arms, interim stopping rules, and other specifications.

Explore
Check out the Health Care Systems Research Collaboratory funded by the National Institutes of Health (https://www.nihcollaboratory.org/Pages/default.aspx). They are involved in collaboration so to improve the design and implementation of clinical trials. Go to their Knowledge Repository and take a look at the types of collaborative projects in which they are involved. Are there some of particular interest to you?

Cluster Randomized Trials

The cluster randomized trial has been advanced as an important study design for comparative effectiveness research. Therapies are randomized and administered at the practice level such as clinics or hospitals instead of at the individual patient level. This is a natural extension of health care in practice. Certain therapies and interventions are usually administered in groups such as various group psychotherapeutic approaches, weight loss classes, and substance abuse programs. Beyond these, there is other natural clustering of health services by location such as wards or units in a hospital, or nursing home residents living in a particular facility that is a part of a large network of facilities. In the hospital setting, interventions may be implemented at the unit level and patient outcomes on each unit can be recorded over time. The hospital itself may constitute a cluster if it is part of a larger consortium of hospitals participating in a study to compare various treatment approaches. These natural clusters—patients within therapy groups, patients within physician practices, hospitals within networks—can form the structural components of a study with a hierarchical design.

The multilevel or cluster design was borrowed from the field of education where the structure of research has historically incorporated basic system elements—students nested within classrooms nested within schools nested within districts. The delivery of health services somewhat mimics this grouping structure.

An example of a cluster randomized trial in a clinical setting was the REDUCE MRSA trial (Randomized Evaluation of Decolonization vs. Universal Clearance to Eliminate Methicillin-Resistant *Staphylococcus aureus*). The results were published in the *New England Journal of Medicine* (Huang, 2013). There were 43 hospitals that participated and the hospitals were randomized to one of three interventions for patients in their intensive care units: (a) screening and isolation; (b) screening, isolation and decolonization of MRSA carriers; or (c) decolonization of all patients without screening. The rates of bloodstream infections were compared and, at the end of the trial, the hospitals that implemented decolonization of all patients without screening (i.e., universal decolonization) had significantly lower rates of bloodstream infection. The universal decolonization approach involved daily bathing of patients with 2% chlorhexidine and the use of the antibiotic mupirocin inside their noses twice daily. The implementation of such cluster randomized trials may have a profound impact on clinical practice in that they can provide strong evidence of benefit or harm in a usual health care setting and do influence practice guidelines.

Stepped Wedge Design. A stepped wedge trial is a type of trial in which the intervention is administered to clusters of patients or providers in a specific time sequence. Randomly assigned clusters are incrementally added over time allowing for sequential enrollment. When implementing a new initiative or service, this allows practitioners to gradually add groups of patients into the study. Because this parallels what often occurs during usual practice, it is a natural choice when considering initiating a new program in health care settings. It also is a natural choice for studies in comparative effectiveness research. For projects using a network of hospitals, each cluster may be a hospital or a group of hospitals. For example, if a patient safety initiative is planned for hospitals nationwide, the hospitals willing to participate are randomized, by sequence, for entry into the study. At the beginning of a stepped wedge trial, baseline measurements are gathered on all hospitals before the start of any interventions. As the trial starts, randomly assigned hospitals enter first and begin the initiative during the first wave. At a later time, another group of hospitals enter and start the intervention (the second wave), and so forth. At the conclusion of the trial during the final wave, all hospitals would be receiving the new intervention. This constitutes a planned phased-in approach. Stepped wedge designs can also be utilized in other health care settings such as primary care clinics, nursing homes, dental clinics, rehabilitation centers, or other settings.

Figure 5.2 displays a visual representation of a typical stepped wedge trial. People are randomized by group or cluster. At the beginning of the trial, no participants are receiving the new therapy (lighter shades). At each point in time, a new cluster is assigned the new therapy (darker shades). At the end of the trial, all clusters are receiving the new therapy. Comparisons of outcomes are made between the times when the new therapy was given versus the outcomes under the older therapy.

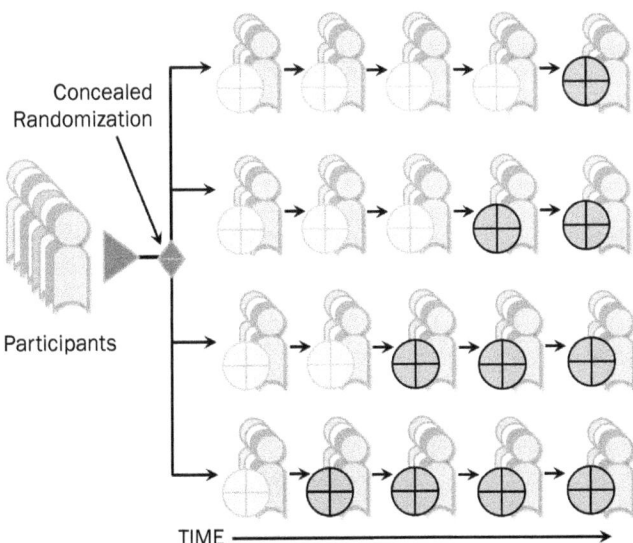

FIGURE 5.2 Randomized Stepped Wedge Trial.

It is important to note that, when feasible, it is valuable to include randomization (by sequence) in a stepped wedge trial. However, in practice, sometimes such interventions are given incrementally over time and randomization to the time of entry for the intervention is not implemented. More careful assessment of baseline differences among the clusters is necessary when studies do not employ randomization.

Crossover Trials

The randomized crossover trial is a design whereby each person in the study receives all of the comparator therapies, and the sequence by which the person receives the therapies is randomized (Figure 5.3). If you are comparing therapy A and therapy B, some patients receive A first, then B. Others receive B first, then A. Individual subjects are randomized to either of the two possible treatment sequences (AB or BA). After receiving each therapy, the patient is assessed for outcome. For a particular patient, he or she would receive therapy A, the outcome would be measured, then receive therapy B, and the outcome would be measured again. The researcher must ensure that the therapy is taken for long enough to expect a particular result and that the outcome is suitable for measurement within the study period.

In a crossover trial, the comparison is within-person. This has some notable advantages. Suppose that we found that functioning improved by 25% with therapy A and 15% with therapy B. The 10% difference in improvement was observed in the same people and therefore, is less likely to be due to extraneous factors. In a crossover trial, matching on the individual is a very powerful way to control for past comorbidities, demographic factors, genetic profile, and past behaviors and exposures (e.g., smoking history, level of physical activity).

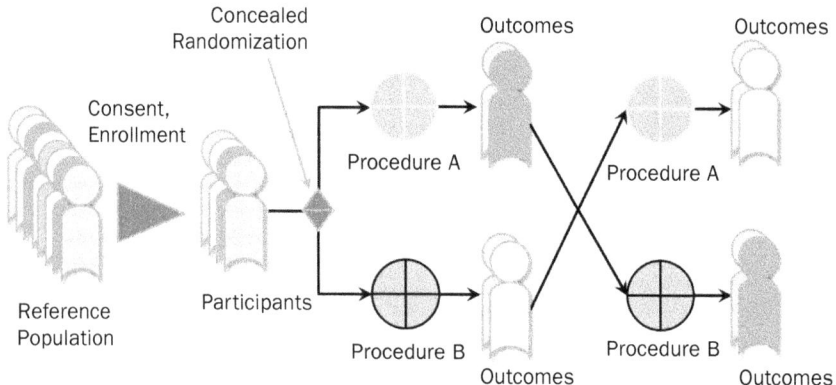

FIGURE 5.3 Randomized Crossover Trial.

We say that such factors are fixed because they remain the same within the individual. Since these factors are constant, differences in episodic events in individuals over time may be more noticeable.

There are a few important issues, however, with crossover trials. In some situations, there could be lingering effects of the therapy over time. What if the patients were still experiencing some of the effects of therapy A when they begin receiving therapy B? The investigator could be measuring some of the combined effects of therapies at the end. We call these carryover effects. Because of such carryover effects, not every therapy can be tested using a crossover trial. One would not likely consider a crossover trial in which major surgery was performed. Therapies that result in permanent changes in the body do not lend themselves to crossover trials. However, for therapies that may be suitable for this approach, the investigator should usually build in a washout period between measurement of the outcome during the first phase and starting the second therapy. This washout period is a time period during which no therapy is given. In drug trials, it is usually a time period in which the drug and its metabolites are excreted by the kidneys before the next drug is given.

> **Think**
> Some outcomes may be suitable for crossover trials while others are not. See if you can think of three outcomes that would not be suitable and three outcomes that could potentially be appropriate for a crossover trial. What common features do they possess?

Another issue that can arise in a crossover trial relates to period effects. Period effects are extraneous impacts on the study results that are not due to the treatments under investigation but rather, to time-related factors correlated with the study variables. Suppose we designed a crossover trial in pregnant women. The women receive one therapy in the second trimester and then a different one in the third trimester. Since there are underlying physiologic differences that are occurring during these two time periods, it may be difficult to tease out true treatment effects from effects that are occurring over the differing trimesters of the pregnancy. A different example would be individuals with progressive chronic conditions such as renal failure. While such conditions do not preclude the use of a crossover trial, one must consider the natural history of the disease itself. However, there may be instances in which the trial would be conducted over a rather short time period, and in such instances, the crossover trial may be an option.

In health care, there is another situation that sometimes occurs which is relevant to the crossover trial. Suppose you intend to compare two different nursing approaches to decreasing the rates of inpatient falls. These approaches are applied at the unit-level of various hospitals within a large network. Units are randomized by treatment sequence (AB or BA), and the nurses apply the appropriate approaches for a two-month period. Fall rates (outcomes) are measured after each treatment with a washout period in-between. But wait a minute. Does something seem different in this trial? The underlying patients in this study are constantly changing. Patients are continually admitted and discharged from the hospital, so instead of the usual within-person comparison that one would expect with a crossover trial, there are different patients receiving A first, then B. And there are different patients receiving B, then A. Welcome to the real world of trying to match a suitable study design to a natural health care setting. Here we have a situation in which the overall structure looks like a cluster crossover trial, but it's not really a within-person comparison. How could we improve upon this design? One tactic would be to realize that a reasonable outcome could be measured at the unit level – say, rate of inpatient falls per 1000 patient-days measured within each unit. The investigator could compare unit outcome rates for each of the nursing procedures. The units would be randomized to the sequence of interventions (procedures) with a washout period between. If the procedures are such that you would expect serious carryover effects, you might also want to consider a stepped wedge design or a conventional randomized trial with multiple comparators in concurrent parallel arms.

N-of-1 Trial

The N-of-1 trial has a natural appeal because it extends what occurs during the ordinary course of life. When you visit your physician, he or she may prescribe a medication based on your symptoms and medical history. You take the drug for a period of time, and if there are appreciable side effects or the desired outcome is not reached, you may contact the physician for reconsideration. Sometimes a different medication is tried, and you see if this one works any better. This trial-within-a-patient is often a mainstay in ordinary practice. This approach, however, can be formalized and restructured, with some additional steps, into an N-of-1 trial. The "N" is a notation for the number of people in the trial, which is one.

Suppose a patient is experiencing chronic, sustained pain and there are two viable options in terms of pain relief—medication A or medication B. Through the assistance of a physician and a pharmacist, this patient could evaluate whether medication A or B is superior (or the same) in terms of pain relief in an N-of-1 trial (Figure 5.4). Since it is possible that knowledge or belief (by the patient or physician) that one of the drugs may be better or worse than the other, it may be wise to incorporate some procedures to minimize this potential bias. Randomization to determine the order of drug administration would occur first (through concealed allocation), and then the sequence (either AB or BA) is blinded to both the patient and the physician throughout the trial. That is, the randomized sequence is generated by an unbiased investigator (sometimes a pharmacist) who conceals the randomization procedure. In addition, the pharmacist ensures that the medications look the same so as to mask the patient and physician to which medication was given at which time.

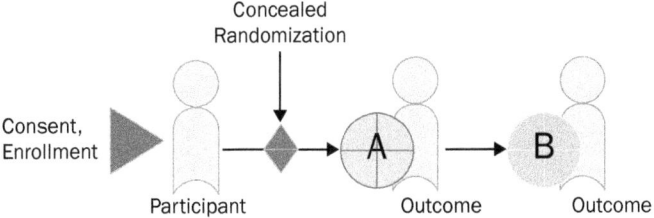

FIGURE 5.4 Randomized N-of-1 Trial.

Note that the concealed randomization procedure (determining whether AB or BA is chosen and keeping this procedure secret) and the blinding (ensuring that the medications look the same) are different, although they are both common design features in trials. If there were three possible medications, the sequence of administration could be randomized as well (ABC or ACB or BCA or BAC or CAB or CBA). The numbers of possible sequence orders are a factorial (n!), so that two medications will yield two random sequences and three medications will yield six random sequences. It is possible to administer the medications repeatedly over time to obtain additional information regarding patient tolerance and pain relief if one expects differing responses over time (e.g., seasons of the year).

Crossover effects should be considered in N-of-1 trials, as in any within-person design. Washout periods can be incorporated so that effects of the first medication would be likely resolved prior to initiation of the second medication. The timing of the washout period should rest on the pharmacological properties of the drug, the anticipated effects in the patient, and practical aspects of study design. For some types of interventions, the washout period may be short (e.g., two days) while for other types of interventions the washout period may be longer (e.g., four months). It is also possible to have interactions among medications, so that the effects of one are amplified or diminished by the presence of another. These concerns should also be considered and could vary depending upon the type of intervention. As always, the choice of comparators is critical. The choices might involve one pain medication versus another, or a particular dose versus a different dose of the same medication.

Most N-of-1 trials include mechanisms for recording several outcomes—the primary endpoint and all secondary endpoints. Both side effects and adverse effects are often recorded. Adverse effects are unwanted or harmful consequences of a medication, while side effects are consequences that are secondary to the intended use of the medication and can be either harmful or beneficial.

Try This
Design an N-of-1 trial in which you would be willing to participate as a patient. Include hypothesis, comparators, outcomes, randomization procedure, blinding, and other details as relevant. Are there certain types of interventions that are more natural fits for an N-of-1 trial? Are there certain interventions that could not easily be answered in an N-of-1 trial?

Factorial Designs

A factorial trial is a method for assessing multiple interventions in the same study. Suppose that you wish to evaluate therapy A versus therapy B, but you don't quite know whether these therapies would be best administered at home or during a clinic visit. You have the comparison of A versus B, but you also have the comparison of home versus clinic. We call the therapies a factor with two levels (A vs. B), and we call the location a factor with two levels as well (home vs. clinic). Hence the name factorial design. We then can assess each possible combination of these factors: A at home, B at home, A at clinic, B at clinic. This particular example would be called a two-by-two factorial design. You could design as many factors and levels as you wish—within limits of feasibility and funding. It is possible to design, for example, a two-by-three factorial design. The two-by-three notation indicates that the first factor has two levels (A, B) and the second factor has three levels (e.g., home, clinic, pharmacy). Keep in mind that as you add more factors and levels within such factors, the additional number of participants required to assess the outcomes would have to be considered.

Within the context of comparative effectiveness research, each of these levels of factors serves as a comparator. In a two-by-two factorial design, there are four comparators. In a two-by-three factorial design, there are six comparators. The researcher then uses such comparators to assess the frequencies of outcomes in each of the study arms. Because of the number of comparisons in this design, the researcher must be careful to consider what the expected frequency of the outcome would be within each of the study arms.

Split-Body Trials

As is readily noticed, humans have bilateral symmetry along the sagittal plane. Our two arms, two legs, two eyes, two ears, two knees, and so forth provide a unique opportunity to assess the effects of treatment on an individual level. This may be particularly germane to topical treatments in which the mirrored body parts are affected, but the choice of therapy is not yet definitive. In this instance, the genetic profile of the patient and most of the important factors that generally impact response (age, gender, current diseases and conditions) are held constant. Therefore, the effects of treatment are more likely to be due to the treatment itself, and the results can be directly beneficial to the participant in the trial. An important consideration, however, is whether the therapy acts locally rather than exhibiting an overall system effect. Split-body trials are utilized for therapies with local effects.

Split body trials can be randomized or not—but the incorporation of randomization adds scientific rigor, and it is relatively straightforward. In addition to randomization, the assessment of outcome can be performed by a practitioner who is blinded to the treatment assignments. If the outcome contains a visual assessment of the appearance of the skin, consider building in a mechanism for masking the person who evaluates and reports the outcome. Make sure that this person does not know which treatment was given on the left or the right side. This will reduce the likelihood of detection bias.

While split-body trials are a within-person comparison, consider enrolling a number of patients into such trials and then reporting the results for an entire group of patients. Sometimes this is useful in finding particular patterns of effectiveness for different types of patients. For example, a therapy may clearly be more effective than another in patients with acute cutaneous lupus erythematosus, but may not be in patients without this condition. This may be an important finding, enhanced by discovery across several patients.

Drug Trials

Testing new drugs involves a series of human trials implemented in phases. Since mediations are such common therapies, knowledge of the general types of scientific studies utilized for testing is valuable. Basic descriptions of such phases are given below:

- **Phase I trials.** First human trial of a drug in a small number of individuals (n = 20–80) to evaluate safety (metabolic effects, toxicity, pharmacologic effects, side effects, dosage).
- **Phase II trials.** Human trial of a drug to first assess likely efficacy with usually 100–300 participants and to further evaluate safety. Metabolic effects, pharmacologic actions, and adverse effects may be assessed.
- **Phase III trials.** Human randomized controlled trial on a large number of participants (n = 1,000–3,000) to assess efficacy of the treatment. Evaluation of overall risk-benefit of treatment and provides data for drug labeling.
- **Phase IV studies.** Postmarketing surveillance of the risks, benefits, and safety issues of a drug after it is introduced into the wider consumer market.

Phase III studies are, perhaps, the most widely known because these large multicenter randomized controlled trials directly assess efficacy as well as safety. The results impact whether the drug will be marketed and used in clinical practice.

Dose Response Trials

A randomized controlled trial that contrasts effects of different doses of a treatment is called a dose-response trial. There may be instances in which a therapy is considered efficacious, and therefore withholding of therapy is considered unethical, but the dose of the therapy may be in question for certain types of patients. Dose response trials are used to evaluate the effects of various drug dosages, although they can be used for other types of comparators as well. An example of a dose response trial of a biologic therapy was a randomized controlled trial conducted using three different doses of platelets to assess degree of bleeding in hospitalized patients with hypoproliferative thrombocytopenia (Slichter, 2010). The investigators found that, for these three specific doses, there were no significant differing effects on the incidence of bleeding in the patients.

For patients in whom quantity of therapies is of appreciable concern such as infants, young children, and older adults, the dose response trial design may be very important. Developmental differences in physiology in the young and pathophysiologic changes due to chronic conditions in older adults may merit investigation due to concerns regarding absorption and excretion of medications. In such instances, dosage may be critical for assessing outcomes while minimizing adverse effects.

Delayed Start Trials

Delayed start trials are studies that can be used to separate symptomology from disease progression. Patients are randomized to either: (a) an early-start group that receives a certain treatment over a fixed time period, or (b) a delayed-start group that receives this treatment at a later point in time. In pharmaceutical trials, a placebo is generally given to group (b) while they are waiting for the active treatment. The ultimate purpose of this design is to determine whether a therapy affects the long-term progression of a chronic disease or whether the therapy provides short-term beneficial effects. Because the main comparison is between people (and not within-person) and the focus is disease progression, it is important that the investigator assess the stage of disease at the onset of the study for all participants or to set enrollment based on a particular stage. For comparative effectiveness research in which the options are viable clinical alternatives, this approach has fewer applications, although there may be select circumstances whereby this approach may be used when a suitable substitute for a placebo is possible.

Equivalence Trials and Noninferiority Trials

Most often, researchers conduct a study to find out if a therapy differs in patient response compared to another therapy. But there are instances in which a researcher may want to determine whether a particular treatment is just as suitable as another—not better and not worse. These may include studies whereby a new therapy is expected to be similar in effect as an established one, but the newer therapy may be less expensive or may be easier for a patient to use (e.g., easier to swallow). Trials to determine that a therapy is not better or worse than another therapy are called equivalence trials. Trials to determine whether a treatment is not worse than another (by a specified margin) are called noninferiority trials.

There are some important considerations in the design of equivalence trials. This relates to the expectation of no difference. What exactly is no difference? For example, how likely is it that the outcome rate would be 13.4/1000 patient-days in therapy A and also 13.4 patient-days in therapy B? Not very likely. Finding the exact same rates is not probable. What if one rate were 13.7/1000 patient-days—would that be close enough? Or what if one of the rates were 14.0/1000 patient-days? That question is what the researcher directly tackles when designing an equivalence trial. How close should close be? This is formally called the equivalence margin. The researcher explicitly sets this difference based on a balance of what is generally considered a clinically important difference and the number of subjects one would need to demonstrate the difference in rates within a given range. Sample size calculations for an equivalence trial are different from those of the usual superiority trials. This is because the hypothesis stipulates a preset difference in rates from one study arm to the other (equivalence margin). We need not go into the calculations here, but be aware that the design for these trials involves different considerations.

Solomon Four Group Design

The Solomon Four Group Design is a traditional trial design that is sometimes used when you expect that the instrument you are using may, in itself, affect the outcome. Applications are more often in educational or behavioral research. The Solomon Four Group design is basically a trial with four groups. Suppose you are a nurse practitioner and you are assessing developmental cognitive measures in preschool children. You plan to compare two behavioral interventions for measuring cognitive abilities (outcome) in two-year-olds. However, you suspect that just by administering the interventions, children may have the opportunity to practice these mental procedures. If you give this intervention once to a child, you suspect that the second time around the child might do a little better. You can assess the effects of the interventions with and without this practice element, so to isolate the effects of the behavioral interventions. In a Solomon Four Group Design, the groups would be set up as such:

> Group 1: Pretest of cognition, intervention A, post-test of cognition
> Group 2: Pretest of cognition, intervention B, post-test of cognition
> Group 3: Intervention A, post-test of cognition
> Group 4: Intervention B, post-test of cognition

The inclusion of groups 3 and 4 (compared to groups 1 and 2) allow the researcher to assess the effects of repeated testing. Note that if only groups 1 and 2 were included, this could mirror a more conventional trial of A versus B. While this more robust trial design would not be customary in comparative effectiveness research, there may be some select instances in which it may be useful.

Preference Trials

In these trials, the patient's preference is taken into consideration when assigning the therapy. As you may imagine, the ultimate preference trial would be to not conduct random assignment. Without randomization, the subjects could decide which therapy they wish to receive. There are preference trials, however, which incorporate some randomization but also feature aspects of patient preference. A few of such designs are described below. Wennberg's design, comprehensive cohort trial design, and Zelen's design are some of the options.

- **Wennberg's design.** The Wennberg trial design first involves randomizing subjects to either a preference group or a randomized group. After this first randomization, the subjects within the preference group are allowed to choose which therapy they would like to receive. The people within the randomized group are then randomized again to each of the comparator therapies. If this were a trial with two comparators (therapy A versus therapy B), the result would yield 4 groups at the end of the study (subjects who chose therapy A, subjects who chose therapy B, subjects who were randomized to therapy A, subjects who were randomized to therapy B). Why design a study in which subjects, who were willing to be randomized at the beginning of the trial, are later allowed to choose treatment? This design is not used often but there may be select instances whereby additional information regarding the effects of the choice of therapy is of interest. These can be compared with the effects without selection bias from the two randomized arms.
- **Comprehensive cohort trial design.** A comprehensive cohort trial is a strategy to address the problems associated with the lack of generalizability in usual randomized controlled trials. In a typical trial, eligible individuals who are not willing to be randomized are not included in the study. Subjects in a typical randomized controlled trial, therefore, may not be as representative of all patients who would be candidates for the treatment in usual practice. By using a comprehensive cohort trial, all persons who are eligible and wish to participate are included (regardless of randomization). Participants who do not wish to be randomized would select their treatment and they would be observed over time similarly as the participants who

were randomized. Both nonrandomized and randomized persons are included in the trial for each of the treatment groups, and outcomes are recorded. This approach could be an option in comparative effectiveness research.
- **Zelen's design.** Another preference trial that incorporates both randomization and preference is the Zelen's design. In the original design, people were randomized prior to obtaining consent. For those randomized to the standard treatment, they would receive it as in usual practice. For those randomized to the new treatment, they would be informed that they were randomized to this new treatment and then given the opportunity to choose whether they wanted it or not. This design poses ethical issues because of the failure to obtain patient consent prior to enrollment and randomization. There are investigators who have implemented modified versions of Zelen's design by addressing the ethical issues regarding patient consent.

Nonrandomized Trials

Many trials can be designed either with or without randomization. If it is unethical or not feasible to randomize, the researcher still has the option of conducting a trial or an intervention study. You can include many of the same elements such as clustering, factorial designs, stepped wedge trials, N-of-1 trials, and crossover trials. All can be performed without the randomization, although the scientific rigor is weakened by doing so. However, in human studies, it is not always possible to randomize because of practical or ethical issues. In fact, nonrandomized interventional studies are quite common in public health.

Trials that are not randomized are sometimes labeled as **quasi-experimental studies**. Such quasi-experimental studies sometimes involve a control group (or a comparator) and sometimes do not. Not all of the quasi-experimental designs are appropriate for comparative effectiveness research because not all involve comparison across two or more treatments. Some suitable controlled designs include the interrupted time series with a comparator which, under some circumstances involve intervention (i.e., an investigator-initiated interrupter), and at other times involve observation only. Quasi-experimental studies without comparators are not suitable designs for comparative effectiveness research, although they may be useful in other disciplines.

Remember that the inability to randomize does not preclude researchers from conducting a trial. Keep in mind the basic definition of a trial. A trial is when an investigator purposefully intervenes during the normal course of life with a particular treatment or intervention in order to assess what occurs afterward. It is this intervention by the researcher that defines a trial—or an experiment.

Why conduct a nonrandomized trial when you could just observe what people naturally do and what occurs in usual clinical practice? A trial necessitates plans for administration of a treatment. A trial has certain advantages because the comparators (i.e., various treatments) can be uniformly applied across all patients. There is more control over how the comparators can be introduced. You can provide additional elements not usually practiced, such as specific educational procedures before and after the comparators are administered. You can structure the study protocol so that, if the comparators involve extended use over time, you can call each subject every two weeks to assess factors related to the intervention. Even without the randomization, a researcher has more control over the administration of the interventions and the follow-up of the subjects than with observation alone. These capabilities can result in more fair comparisons between different therapies. Some may argue that by using a trial you would not be assessing the comparators in a real-world situation. While this is true, new health services and initiatives often involve staff and patient education anyways and, by giving this some structure, you are ensuring that the comparators are delivered in a uniform manner across the study groups. Thus, nonrandomized trials of comparators constitute a suitable option for comparative effectiveness research.

Natural Experiments

There are instances that occasionally occur in populations in which exposures are distributed differently among groups of people and, because of this natural distribution, one can see patterns of different outcomes in the population. People receiving a certain service may have better outcomes, while people receiving a different service have poorer outcomes. An oft-cited example of a natural experiment deals with the grouping of Londoners by water district in the 1800s. By virtue of the water district, the rates of cholera differed. John Snow carefully delineated differences in cholera death rates by water district. The water districts served as the natural comparators, since contamination of the water with *Vibrio cholerae* varied by district. This was quite the discovery, since the germ theory of infectious disease had not yet been developed. This natural experiment formed the basis of early epidemiology.

Enactment of laws or policies at a regional level may sometimes produce effects that could be considered natural experiments. If, in one region, there are higher taxes on tobacco products, tobacco use may decrease which then improves health. The health of populations across regions with differing taxes can be compared. In this case it isn't the tax that physiologically causes illness, but the tax influences the use of tobacco products (which then impact health). It is through this pathway that the tax ultimately influences health. Some scientists call these third factors (such as the tobacco tax or the water district in the examples above) **instrumental variables**.

Experimentation Versus Observation

Trials involve experimentation. They can provide important information regarding choices that have relevance in decision making. But experiments are not the only venue available in science. The scientific method involves two core processes—experimentation and observation. Observation can also be instructive, and can provide evidence of natural occurrences. There will probably never be a randomized controlled trial of vision and driving an automobile. There will be no randomization of people who need eyeglasses to either wearing their eyeglasses/contacts or not wearing them, and then assessing their driving abilities. We do not need a trial to know that people who are legally blind without their eyeglasses should not be driving a car without them. Why do we know this? Observation. In fact, this is so evident through observation that in many places (but not all!), you must pass a vision test before receiving a driver's license.

> **Explore**
> Instrumental variables are becoming increasing utilized in comparative effectiveness research. Some people use instrumental variables (or instruments) as natural randomizers. The water district served as a natural randomizer for people living in London in the 1800s at the time of the cholera outbreaks. The tobacco tax in certain areas served as a natural randomizer affecting tobacco sales, which then affected health outcomes. Both of these instruments had a geographical dimension. By virtue of where people lived, they were exposed to different factors. Go online to PubMed Central to find other examples of instrumental variables. There is a review study by Brookhart and colleagues entitled, "Instrumental Variable Methods in Comparative Safety and Effectiveness Research" (http://www.ncbi.nlm.nih.gov/pmc/articles/PMC2886161/). Scroll down the article until you find, "Examples of Instrumental Variables in Healthcare Research." Take a look at the variety of different instruments used.

> **Scientific observation** involves the sensing of occurrences and the recording of what occurred in a detailed, consistent, and unbiased manner, with an *a priori* protocol of what to record and when to record it.

Observational studies are of greatest impact when the differences in therapies are very noticeable in everyday life. One such example occurred through observations of young women. It was a case-control study with only eight cases—young women who had developed adenocarcinoma of the vagina (Herbst, 1971). Seven of these eight young women had a mother who had taken diethylstilbestrol during pregnancy, but none of the mothers of the controls did. Even though there had been clinical trials of diethylstilbestrol conducted before this case-control study, the difference was so stark that it changed practice.

There are some observational studies in which subjects are actively enrolled in real-time and are observed over a specific time period. These are prospective studies. Sometimes there is a record of therapies and health-related events that are already captured in electronic databases, and the investigator

> **Discover**
> There have been several large prominent cohort studies conducted in various countries. The Framingham Heart Study is one. Take a look at it online (http://www.framinghamheartstudy.org/). What types of important information did we learn from the Framingham Heart Study? Can you name any other well-known cohort studies?

needs only to go to these databases to extract the information to complete a study. These are retrospective studies. For both prospective and retrospective approaches, there are various designs.

There are a number of reasons why randomized trials cannot always answer important questions that patients may have. One is that most randomized trials do not contain a sufficient number and variety of people in order to adequately evaluate all beneficial, adverse, and side effects of therapies. Sometimes adverse effects are rather uncommon, or they may occur in certain types of people, and therefore, the effects may not be evident without data on large populations.

Randomized trials can demonstrate short-term effects but may not provide adequate information for evaluating long-term effects, particularly those that occur 10 or 20 years into the future. Large, comprehensive longitudinal databases of individuals receiving treatments over extended periods of time are often necessary to assess such effects. Long-term effects of many medications, in particular, are not fully known, especially for individuals with multiple comorbidities and who are taking a variety of different drugs. However, observational pharmacovigilance studies can be quite informative in this respect.

Observational designs may also be a viable option for rapidly evolving technologies. Observational person-level registries of devices or technologies may serve an important function through real-time detection of potential issues related to utilization and safety. Tracking patients' responses over time with the use of certain devices or services may be an important compliment to randomized trials.

When conducting observational research, we use several criteria to help discern whether the effect is due to differences among the viable comparators and not some extraneous factor.

- When the difference in treatment effect is very large between one therapy and another, we are more likely to say that it is not due to chance.
- If several researchers looked at the therapies in slightly different ways in many studies but they all showed a consistent effect, the results are more likely to be true.
- In some instances, when there is a dose-response in which an increasing amount of the therapy leads to an increased probability of the outcome, we are more likely to believe the effect.
- If the totality of the evidence with animal studies, physiologic studies, and pharmacologic studies all support the findings from observational studies, one is more likely to say that the results are valid.

- If the study incorporates ways to control for potential extraneous factors that may be artificially influencing the pathways under investigation, one is more likely to believe the results.
- If the researchers definitively demonstrated the temporal sequence of events so that the patient outcomes occurred after the onset of therapy, the results would support a potential causal effect.

One approach to demonstrating effect is to use within-person comparisons. Let's start with an examination of some within-person observational designs and then explore some between-person options.

Case-Crossover Studies and Self-Controlled Case Series

There is no better match than oneself. Everyone has a unique genetic profile and medical history. In a within-person design, the researcher uses this match and exploits opportunities when events occur at different times. A person may be taking a particular medication for several years and then, after switching to a new medication, a blood clot occurs. In these designs, the researcher can investigate what happened just prior to an acute event (blood clot) and then compare this to what usually occurs at other times. What medications or other therapies was the patient using just prior to the blood clot? How does this compare to the mediations and therapies that the patient used at other times? For these studies, the investigators must have dates or time-relevant data to calculate times when exposures and outcomes occurred, which may be available in large clinical databases. Such designs can be very powerful in controlling for potential confounding factors. In fact, the degree of matching is even stronger than the equivalency found through randomization of different people to various treatment groups in trials.

This type of design, however, is only suitable for particular types of exposures and outcomes. The outcomes must be acute events and the exposures (or therapies) must exhibit variability or have the potential to change over time within the same person. Sometimes these exposures can be thought of as triggers of an acute event. Heavy lifting, being angry, sexual activity, or having an infection have all been implicated as triggers of acute myocardial infarction. These were discovered through with-person comparative designs. Sometimes immediate effects of treatment are also great candidates for within-person designs. Examinations of effects after vaccination have been conducted using within-person comparisons with good success. The time period after vaccination can be compared with other time periods in the same individual.

There are several observational designs that utilize within-person comparisons. These include case-crossover studies and self-controlled case series.

¤ **Case-crossover studies.** In these studies, an investigator observes the exposures or therapies that occurred prior to an outcome event and uses other time periods as the comparators for determining the background or usual frequency of such occurrences (Figure 5.5). A case-crossover study begins with the selection of the time of the acute event (outcome) for each participant. For example, this may be the dates when pulmonary embolism occurred in a patient population. Or it could be ischemic stroke, epileptic seizure, a fractured rib, or other injuries. The onset of the outcome must be definable. This information can originate from databases in which dates of events are recorded. If we have reason to believe that the exposures under investigation exert their effects within 1 week, then we could use a 7-day at-risk window prior to the acute event. The next step is to select other time windows when the outcome did not occur. The frequency of exposures (illustrated by A in Figure 5.5) can be determined in the multiple comparison time windows and this frequency can be compared to the exposure frequency just before the acute event. So, for example, were patients more likely to receive erythropoiesis-stimulating agents just prior to their pulmonary embolism compared to other time periods?

Variants of the case-crossover design can also be used for episodes of health care. For example, one application would be to use a particular hospitalization for a patient and match this with other hospitalizations for the same patient. Suppose, during one hospitalization, the patient developed a serious infection—a *Clostridium difficile* infection. However, this patient had subsequent hospitalizations over the next three years in which no *Clostridium difficile* infection occurred. The question becomes, "Why did this patient develop this infection during this one hospitalization but not in the others?" The investigator then examines what occurred in the hospital just prior to the *Clostridium difficile* infection (time at risk) and compares this with what occurred during the other hospitalizations. Therapies and procedures given during the time at risk would be of interest.

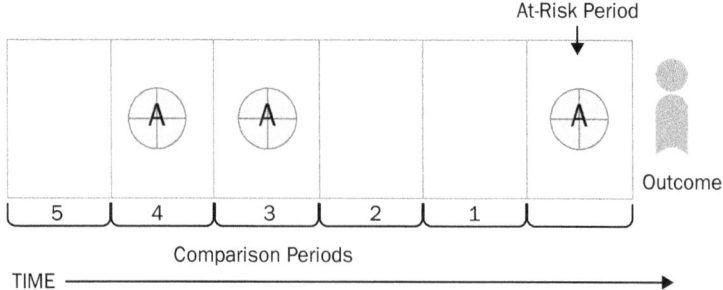

FIGURE 5.5 Design of a Case-Crossover Study.

Another robust within-person design is the self-controlled case series.

- **Self-controlled case series.** The design of the self-controlled case series is slightly different from the case-crossover study. Similar to the case-crossover study, only cases (people with acute events) are included. However, in the self-controlled case series, the investigator starts with the timing of the exposure and develops the risk periods when the subjects were exposed and uses the other time periods as the control or comparison periods. The researcher then determines the incidence rate of the acute event (outcome) during the exposure periods and the incidence rate of the outcome during the comparison periods.

These designs work well for studies in which a new drug, biologic, or service is being introduced to the general public at large. The frequency of specific outcomes can be compared for the new drug versus the patient's history with an existing treatment.

Often within-person comparator studies derive their information from an existing large medical database or linked databases. That is, the studies are retrospective in that all the information regarding the therapies and outcomes already occurred. However, there have been case-crossover studies of patients with acute events in which the prior exposures were ascertained from patient recall. Not all retrospective databases have detailed data regarding the types of triggers of interest such as sexual activity or stressful events. Sometimes only the patient can provide such information. Disadvantages are that only survivors are available for the recall and that memory itself may be influenced by the event.

There are some questions in which within-person comparisons work very well, but there are other instances in which this approach must be critically evaluated prior to selection. If the therapy under investigation leads to permanent changes in an individual (e.g., removal of an organ), then the comparison time periods cannot include the time after the permanent change took place. If the outcome is not sudden but occurs slowly over the course of years (e.g., in the case of slow growing tumors), the case-crossover study may not be an option. However, for the ascertainment of episodic therapies and acute events, these within-person studies are important tools for comparative effectiveness research.

Longitudinal Designs

Longitudinal observational designs are anticipated to be important contributors to comparative effectiveness research. Such studies may involve investigations using massive electronic databases in which populations are observed over time and in which detailed clinical data are available to answer meaningful questions. These are retrospective designs. Alternatively, prospective longitudinal studies can also be conducted to collect the types of information relevant for specific therapies and to capture patient-reported outcomes.

For most seasoned researchers, one cannot overemphasize the importance of being able to examine what occurs to people longitudinally – as they move from health to each medical diagnosis and with each medical procedure. To date, it has been difficult for researchers to capture the complexity of peoples' lives so that there are meaningful expectations of events over lifespans. Hopefully, the methods of prediction and the data available to generate such predictions will advance. To be clear, the simple linking of an independent variable (a therapy) with a single dependent variable (an outcome), as the most common paradigm in published medical studies, doesn't go far enough. I encourage you, as a researcher, to explore ways in which we can find avenues to take longitudinal data and provide meaningful answers in our complex lives.

Common types of longitudinal studies include interrupted time series with comparators, cohort studies, and panel studies.

Interrupted Time Series with Comparators

Interrupted time series is a longitudinal design in which group-level measures are repeatedly collected over a specific time period and, during the time period, there was a change in policy or service (the "interrupter"). The magnitude of the change in group-level measures is compared in the time period before and after the interrupter. When available, these data are contrasted to other sites or regions in which the interrupter did not occur; this constitutes an interrupted time series with an external comparator. An interrupted time series can be utilized without a comparator—with the basic before and after comparison—but, from the perspective of comparative effectiveness research, either an internal comparator (another service at the same site) or an external comparator (another service at other sites) would be preferable. This external comparator is often used to measure temporal or background outcome rates that occur without the interrupter.

Figure 5.6 illustrates the results from an interrupted time series design, showing measurements of the outcome (e.g., complication rates) over time in the group that receives the new treatment (dark lines) and the comparator group (grey lines).

While interrupted time series can be used in research, it also has extensive applications in quality control initiatives in health care and patient safety surveillance. For example, you may have access to early elective delivery rates (prior to 39 weeks gestation) and these rates are measured each month across

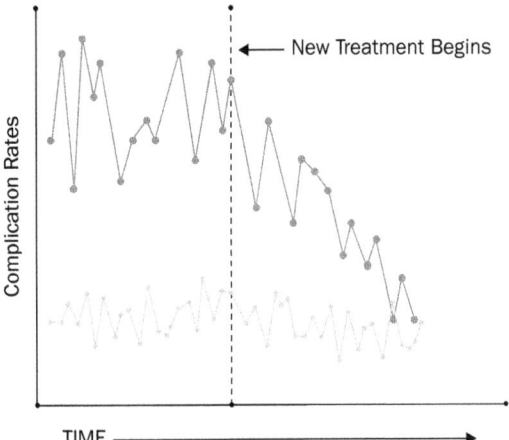

FIGURE 5.6 Interrupted Time Series with Comparator.

a network of hospitals. You measure monthly elective delivery rates for 12 consecutive months. You apply a new prevention initiative across some of the hospitals, but do not in the others. You then measure elective delivery rates for 12 months afterward. That is the basic structure of an interrupted time series. There is a series of "before" measurements (the rates before the prevention initiative), the intervention commenced, and then a series of "after" monthly rates. In the hospitals without the initiative, there is a series of measurements of monthly elective delivery rates across the entire time period. Most often, a new initiative occurring in some hospitals is compared with standard practice (defined) in the other hospitals. However, the investigator could compare two different prevention initiatives if desired –one initiative in some hospitals and another initiative in the other hospitals. Of note, hospitals across the United States are actively working to end elective deliveries prior to 39 weeks gestation unless medically necessary. Part of these prevention policies address patient education regarding the risks associated with early elective inductions.

There are also wider applications in the general population. Suppose that in several communities you collected annual suicide rates in young adults over the past 20 years. In one of the communities, a school-based suicide prevention program was instituted 10 years ago. In another community, a primary care provider-based suicide prevention program was instituted at a similar time. A researcher can use this information to conduct comparative effectiveness research. There is a comparison between the suicide rates before and after each prevention program, but there is also the comparison between the suicide rates in the community with the school-based intervention versus the provider-based intervention. One could answer the following questions. In comparison to the suicide rates before the programs occurred, did the suicide rates change after each of these interventions? If so, by how much? Were the rates of change after the program started any different for the school-based program versus the provider-based program, with adjustment for baseline rates? These results can provide very valuable information so as to direct community efforts to the program that better achieves the desired outcomes.

Sometimes, the intervention (or interrupter) in this design is not explicitly manipulated by the researcher, but was something that occurred as a part of routine clinical practice or was initiated because of a new program or health policy (unrelated to research purposes). Such health policies can be utilized as opportunities to conduct comparative effectiveness research studies. Did the health policy affect patient-relevant outcomes? With the advent of the changes in the health care laws within the United States, the variability in Medicaid coverage, in particular, can be utilized to explore differences in peoples' health from state to state using such interrupted time series approaches. States with similar coverage policies can be compared to states that chose other options. Before and after comparisons can be made, as well as contrasts among the states. This may be a unique opportunity to investigate important patient outcomes through variation in policies.

Such interrupted time series designs work well for events that are routinely recorded over time—regardless of whether a research study was initially planned. One example for population-based measures would be disease surveillance, usually conducted by agencies such as the Centers for Disease Control and Prevention or the World Health Organization. When conducting hospital-based studies, often event measures are evaluated for purposes of patient safety, including injuries and infection rates. Such routine surveillance can serve as a starting point for designing an interrupted time series design.

The interrupters can be any treatment, service, or policy. It can even be a natural disaster, such as an earthquake that occurred in one location but not another, or a hurricane or a wildfire. How did these disasters affect emergency services and patient outcomes? The interrupted time series design may be an important approach to evaluate population responses to natural disasters. There are many options depending upon your area of investigation. There may be a targeted media campaign related to health education in several areas that did not occur in other regions. The health effects of this "interrupter" may be compared with occurrences prior to its initiation, and these can be contrasted to health outcomes in the regions without such a campaign.

Check It Out
Go to the Web-based Injury Statistics Query and Reporting System in the Injury Prevention & Control section at the Centers for Disease Control and Prevention (http://www.cdc.gov/injury/wisqars/index.html). Select "nonfatal injury data" and choose Nonfatal injury 2001–2011. You can obtain data for each of these specific years by various characteristics. Make yourself a time series with some of the options of interest to you. For example, you can see whether or not the rates of injuries by BB or pellet guns have changed from 2001 to 2011.

Trend Studies in General. The interrupted time series with comparators is a type of design within a larger rubric of trend studies.

In trend studies, data regarding a population are collected over time, but the sample taken from the population may be different at each assessment in time. These studies track trends in the underlying population over time but do not necessarily sample the same people at each assessment. Comparisons regarding utilization and patient outcomes can be made across geographic regions. In addition, such information may be utilized in decision analyses. An example of these types of data involves trend information available through the Healthcare Cost and Utilization Project (http://www.ahrq.gov/research/data/hcup/index.html). In this project, information is collected from hospitals in various states each year. The participating hospitals and patients within the hospitals may change from one year to the next. Trend analyses can be performed to investigate time-related changes or similarities in health-relevant events in the entire reference population.

Check It Out
If you would like to see quick statistics on hospitals, check out HCUPnet (http://hcupnet.ahrq.gov/). This is a publicly available query system in which you can obtain information on hospitals and emergency departments. When you come to the main page, select National Statistics on All Stays. On the next screen, go ahead and select Researcher, Medical Professional. Notice that one of the options is Trends. Select any type of data for which you would like to see trends over time. Explore. See how each measure changes. Feel free to investigate other options available at the HCUPnet site. There is more information readily available than just trends.

Trend analyses are quite common when conducting quality control initiatives in health care settings. Rates of infection, such as central venous catheter-related bloodstream infection rates, can be tracked over time at a given hospital or over a network of hospitals. Within the medical community, there is a collection of patient safety indicators that are monitored over time. Besides infection, they include complications such as a foreign body left during a procedure, birth trauma rates, accidental punctures or laceration rates, and other measures. Often these measures are reported routinely over time, and the results are displayed by trend analyses. Such measures usually do not track or reflect specific patients over time, but from a given source population, they assess the same indices routinely over time. Sometimes such patient safety indicators form the basis of published medical research studies.

Cohort Studies

A cohort is a defined group of people with shared characteristics who are observed over a period of time. Based on study objectives, a cohort study involves defining the participants in the study, collecting baseline data on such individuals, observing and recording their use

Discover
Search for Patient Safety Indicators (http://www.qualityindicators.ahrq.gov/modules/psi_resources.aspx) or the Patient Safety Network (http://psnet.ahrq.gov/default.aspx), and you will find the list of the indicators online. What types of patient safety indicators are there? If you were to suggest an additional patient safety indicator, what would it be?

of various therapies or exposures during the study period, and then observing such people over time for the incidence of the outcomes. At the start of the study, information is collected regarding subject characteristics and other factors relevant to the investigation. Historically, subjects were defined initially by their exposure or use of a certain therapy (e.g., a specific physical activity regimen) and outcomes would be examined in those individuals who adhered to this regimen and compared to individuals who did not. However, there are variations on the design elements such that exposures can vary and be measured over time (time-varying exposures). In addition, the outcomes can be measured uniformly at a fixed time period, say 60 days after enrollment, yielding a cumulative risk of the outcome in various subjects. Alternatively, the outcomes can be measured such that the metric of interest is the time until the subjects experienced the outcome (time to event analyses). So, although we may be observing this collective group of people over time within the context of the cohort study, there are several variations in design available to the researcher. At the end of the investigation one generally wishes to make inferences about a wider population, so there should be careful thought regarding how to select the participants and who they represent, so that proper inferences can be made at the conclusion of the study.

Cohort studies can be retrospective or prospective. In comparative effectiveness research, retrospective approaches using large electronic clinical databases of longitudinal populations can be valuable. Databases can be utilized from health insurers, providers, federal agencies, or from pre-existing longitudinal studies. Increasingly, databases are being linked to broaden the types of information available or to enhance the depth of clinical data.

The availability of electronic health data—from medical records, research studies, health insurers, governmental surveys and through other mechanisms—indicates that there will be considerable opportunities for research in the near future. Many of these databases are broad and multipurpose and therefore, they are not structured just for a particular hypothesis-driven research study.

Explore

There are increasingly more consortia and networks that have integrated longitudinal databases. Look at the Netherland Information Network of General Practice (http://www.nivel.nl/en/netherlands-information-network-general-practice-linh). They have a longitudinal clinical database. How many individuals are in this database? What general types of information do they house? Also look at the EU-ADR project (http://www.euadr-project.org/). How many people are in their database? What types of information do they collect? Also look at the Health Improvement Network (http://epi.grants.cancer.gov/pharm/pharmacoepi_db/thin.html). How many patients are in their system and types of data are available? You might also want to explore the linked databases available through the Surveillance Epidemiology and End Results program (http://seer.cancer.gov/resources/ linked_databases.html) as well. There are an increasing number of large, potentially valuable longitudinal clinical databases to explore. See if you can find others with information online.

Rather, the data are extensive and the onus is on the researcher to structure the variables into a meaningful design. Historically, cohort studies were of two types: (a) cohorts formed from one common population whereby those individuals exposed to a certain factors were compared to those who were not exposed within the same cohort and (b) cohorts in which a group of people exposed to a factor were compared to an external group not exposed. Often, the external comparison was of individuals from different working environments exposed to different workplace factors, as in occupational medicine. However, external comparators can be utilized in other settings as well. With large electronic databases on populations, the exposed and unexposed can be extracted from the same database so that external comparators need not always be necessary. However, it is possible that instances may arise whereby external comparators would find a use.

In another example, pregnancy forms a natural cohort. Women who are pregnant could be observed from early pregnancy through the postpartum period (as they often are in practice). Inception cohorts are those in which people are assembled close to the onset of their exposure or services of interest. As an example, this could be at the time of the first prenatal visit when a new eHealth application is being evaluated to promote better adherence to health behaviors during the pregnancy (compared to simpler printed materials). Outcomes could be related to the health status or functioning of the expectant mother or the health status of the newborn at the time of or after delivery.

Discover
Some types of individuals naturally form a cohort. Perhaps the most common are birth cohorts. The National Children's Study is following more than 100,000 children in the United States from before birth until age 21 to study environmental effects, health, and development (http://www.nationalchildrensstudy.gov/Pages/default.aspx). Take a look at the types of information that they intend to collect. The Millenium Cohort Study in the United Kingdom is an example in which approximately 19,000 infants born in 2000-2001 are being followed over time to assess child and parental health as well as other developmental, social, and educational factors. You can follow their progress at the Centre for Longitudinal Studies (http://www.cls.ioe.ac.uk/page.aspx?&sitesectionid=851&sitesectiontitle=Welcome+to+the+Millennium+Cohort+Study). Other cohorts are assembled based on occupation. One large well-known study is the Nurses' Health Study, which originated with a cohort of over 120,000 female registered nurses, with additional assemblages of large cohorts in the ensuing years (http://www.channing.harvard.edu/nhs/). Evaluation of risk factors for chronic diseases was one of the principal goals, with dietary assessment constituting a large component of the study. Check out some of their findings. Another well-known occupational cohort was the British Doctors Study, which began back in 1951 and generated studies showing a link between smoking and lung cancer. Any occupational group—accountants or salon workers or airline attendants—could form the foundation of a cohort if they were willing and mechanisms for building informational databases were in place. If you were to start a longitudinal cohort, what types of people would you enroll? Why?

Other natural cohorts include members of the armed forces in which health status over time can be monitored. In the United States, the Millenium

Cohort Study is a longitudinal study of US military personnel (not to be confused with the cohort of the same name in the United Kingdom) in which almost 150,000 people are being observed.

Sometimes the cohort involves a group of individuals who have common experiences: for example, alumni who graduated from a particular university in a particular year. The group can be members of a particular registry—a cancer registry or diabetes registry. Or the group can be members of a weight-loss program, a meditation group, or a smoking cessation program. They could also be members of a particular social interest group that can be assessed over time via the Web. For comparative effectiveness research, it is often helpful if the group is already monitored over time by health professionals. Then information regarding baseline characteristics—and sometimes health-relevant exposures, events, and outcomes—may already be available.

Practice-Based Evidence for Clinical Practice Improvement. An umbrella term for various observational study designs within comparative effectiveness research has been defined as practice-based evidence for clinical practice improvement (Horn, 2007). The characteristics of practice-based evidence studies have been described and mirror those of pragmatic studies including relevance to clinical practice, diverse study participants and practices, and the measurement of many relevant outcomes (Tunis, 2003). Often the designs utilized for practice-based evidence studies are longitudinal in nature and follow a prospective cohort design, although other longitudinal designs (panel studies, trend studies) may have applications as well. For patients with specific conditions, practice-based evidence designs strive to include all therapies relevant to the condition under investigation, have generalized hypotheses with more inclusive selection criteria, employ measures of illness severity and functional status, utilize statistical control to address baseline patient differences rather than randomization, and include a transdisciplinary Clinical Practice Team and transparency for stakeholders (Horn, 2007).

Panel Studies

Another longitudinal design is the panel study. In panel studies, a sample is drawn from a population, and surveys are repeatedly collected from the sample over time. The sample is often people or households. Observations are recorded, generally through self-report on questionnaires or through interviews. The sample is called a panel, and each time at which the surveys or interviews are collected is called a wave. For example, households may be sampled from the entire population during 2004 and one adult in the household is chosen to answer questions regarding the members of the household. These households are then observed every two years for 10 years. Interviews during year 2004 constitute the first wave, interviews during year 2006 constitute the second wave, and so forth. Repeated measures are taken on these specific households. In some studies, it is only the households that were selected at the beginning of the study and are then followed; thus, it is the same household observed throughout the entire study period. This actually could be classified as a cohort study in which the same people (or a defined group of people) are observed over time. In some panel studies, however, new people or groups of people (e.g., households) may enter during the course of the study. So, for example, in 2008 other households might be added to the original sample of households. Panel studies have several variations that relate to the recruitment of new subjects and the retention of persons from earlier waves. If the unit of observation in a panel study is a household or a family, care must be taken to define such entities for purposes of the study. During ordinary life, households tend to be fluid with family members and residents moving in and out. Thus, various *a priori* rules are set regarding definitions before the onset of the panel study.

Panel studies that utilize repeated surveys are more common in the social sciences, but are sometimes utilized in health-related research as well. For example, the Health and Retirement Study is a panel study in which the participants are interviewed every two years for the same information regarding retirement, health, and finances. Sometimes additional information is added as well. Other types of data have been linked to the Health and Retirement Study, such as Medicare files and the National Death Index. Some of the health-related information, then, originates in the biennial interviews, and other health-related data can be extracted from the files obtained through linking databases. Information from the Centers for Medicare and Medicaid Services includes files with information regarding hospital stays, skilled nursing facility stays, outpatient visits including physician visits and other Medicare-approved providers, visits to emergency departments, short stays in ambulatory surgical centers, home health visits, and hospice care. This information includes the dates of services and the types of services received, including procedures, the diagnoses of the patient, and other data. Such information provides a descriptive pattern of medical care received over an extensive period of time, and when combined with the biennial interviews that capture demographic information and health-related behaviors, these databases can be utilized to provide answers to many research questions.

Panel studies are common throughout the world. Examples include the German

---

Take A Look
The longest running panel study began in 1968 and constitutes a nationally representative sample of over 18,000 people. It is called the Panel Study of Income Dynamics. Search for it online (http://psidonline.isr.umich.edu/). While you are at the Institute for Social Research, also check out their Health and Retirement Study. At their main page (http://hrsonline.isr.umich.edu/), click on Concordance. You will see a list of sections within the data sets. Select one of the options within the Health section and see what pops up. You can see each question that was asked regarding a particular topic.

Socio-Economic Panel, which began in 1984; the British Household Panel Survey, which started in 1991; the European Community Household Panel, which started in 1994; and the Household and the Income and Labour Dynamics in Australia Survey, which began in 2001.

Longitudinal Databases

Health care systems that have integrated longitudinal data across an entire population provide opportunities for investigating effectiveness of therapies and services. For comparative effectiveness research, population-based data can serve as a valuable sampling frame. For example, one could obtain data regarding all individuals receiving specific therapies, and then observe outcomes through time. Or the entire population could be observed for variations in outcome effects across different exposures.

Databases for longitudinal studies suitable for comparative effectiveness research may originate from various sources, including the following:

- **Public health databases.** Many governments conduct longitudinal surveys for public health purposes. Examples of such databases can be found online at the Centers for Disease Control and Prevention Public-Use Data Files and Documentation site (http://www.cdc.gov/nchs/data_access/ftp_data.htm). These databases are freely available for research purposes. Information regarding linked files can be found at the National Center for Health Statistics Data Linkage Activities (http://www.cdc.gov/nchs/data_access/data_linkage_activities.htm).
- **Health insurance databases.** Longitudinal patient-specific information is sometimes available through claims from health insurers, whether public or private. Examples are data files available from the Centers for Medicare and Medicaid Services in the United States (http://www.resdac.org/cms-data). Other large health insurers such as Kaiser Permamente conduct clinical research as well (http://www.dor.kaiser.org/external/research/topics/Medical_Informatics/).
- **Databases from health care providers**. Hospitals, hospital consortiums, networks of physician practices, and other providers may serve as a source of electronic medical records for patient-level data. The University HealthSystem Consortium is one example (https://www.uhc.edu/home.htm). They have several medical databases appropriate for comparative effectiveness research.
- **Databases of longitudinal studies**. There have been many longitudinal studies that were conducted by teams of researchers, usually in academia. Often such studies were federally funded. Sometimes these databases are available for other researchers to use.

An example is the Framingham Heart Study and the Health and Retirement Study.
- ¤ **Databases generated through registries**. Registries can be an important source of data for investigation. Some registries are disease-based, while others related to specific products, medical devices, or drugs. An example of a disease-based linked registry is the Surveillance, Epidemiology, and End Results (SEER) program of cancer registries funded through the National Cancer Institute, which has been linked with Medicare data (http://healthservices.cancer.gov/seermedicare/). Patients are observed from the time of Medicare eligibility until death.

Discover

The Research Data Assistance Center (ResDAC) provides training and resources for researchers who work with data from the Centers for Medicare and Medicaid Services. ResDAC can be very helpful in learning what information is available, how to obtain the files, and how to work with the data. Search for ResDAC online (http://www.resdac.org/) and look at the documentation for the various data files. Next, try searching for the Chronic Conditions Data Warehouse (http://www.ccwdata.org). This is a database with longitudinal data regarding medical services received through Medicare and Medicaid in the United States. Data are available regarding hospitalizations, emergency department visits, skilled nursing facility visits, doctor office visits, other clinic visits, home health visits, medical equipment utilized, and prescription drugs. If you would like a quick look at some data, try their Chronic Conditions Dashboard. You can see the prevalence of various chronic conditions, spending by condition and age, gender-specific information, and geographic information. Does anything surprising pop up?

Case-Control Designs

Case-control studies are common in the medical literature, but are often utilized for hypothesis generation rather than studies of effectiveness. In a case-control study, people with a given condition or outcome (cases) are first selected. Then controls are chosen based on the hypotheses being tested, the characteristics of the cases, and considerations relevant to the reference population of interest. As a general principle, the controls should be drawn from the population from which the cases arose. Population-based case-control studies tend to be the more robust in design when (a) cases comprise all those people who developed the disease in a certain geographical region during a specific time period, and (b) controls are a representative or random sample of the underlying population in the region during the same time period.

In clinical research, it is more common to observe case-control studies that are based on patients (cases) seen in a medical setting (e.g., physician's office, hospital), and controls are other patients are that same environment. In a typical case-control study, the most important design feature is the selection of the control or comparison group. This is the group that will form the frequencies for comparisons. In health care settings such as hospitals, the comparison groups generally tend to be patients who are being treated for conditions other than that of interest in the study. Sometimes this collective group may be difficult to describe when captured across hospitals, because often hospitals specialize in certain types of services and this influences the types of patients admitted. When choosing this design, always ask yourself what types of patients will constitute the comparison and how this may affect the interpretation of the results. The more robust alternatives in these settings involve those designs in which cases represent all such individuals with a condition within a large service network that serves a defined population. Controls could be selected from those individuals who also receive their health care within the same network.

When the data are all electronic, however, often the choice of a longitudinal design is preferable, which enables the researcher to directly calculate the outcome risks in each study group. However, there may be selected circumstances in which a case-control design would be utilized in comparative effectiveness research. For example:

- **Personalized medicine studies.** In studies where DNA testing is an integral part of the design and the researcher is interested in a particular clinical outcome, the case-control study can be a reasonable approach. For example, cases could be patients who do not find allergy relief from a certain allergy medication (nonresponders), and they are asked to submit a DNA sample for testing. Controls can be patients with similar clinical profiles who also receive the allergy drug but, for these individuals, they do find relief from their allergy symptoms (responders). They also are asked to submit a DNA sample. This particular case-control study is not a head-to-head comparison of therapies, but the information from this study could be used to design a head-to-head comparative study of possible allergy medications in nonresponders.
- **Studies of rare conditions.** There are rare disease registries that can serve as a starting point for a case-control study. When data regarding individuals' responses to various therapies are available, this may provide an opportunity to assess whether the symptoms or level of functioning improve for certain therapies compared to others. If the researcher begins with a defined group of cases (e.g., patients who, given their stage of disease, are functioning poorly), such patients can be compared to individuals with this disease at the same stage who are functioning well. Are there differences in the therapies that distinguish those patients who are functioning well from those who are not? Sometimes such case-control studies do not have the ability to find differences because of small sample sizes, but occasionally, if a therapy or a service is very beneficial (or very detrimental), such effects can be seen.

Information generated from case-control designs is often utilized within a body of evidence relevant for a particular hypothesis prior to the development of trials. Well-designed, population-based case-control studies can be useful in this role.

Twin Studies

Many studies of twin siblings have been conducted to sort out the degree to which events are likely to be due to genetic versus environmental factors. A common approach is to compare identical (monozygotic) twin pairs with fraternal (dizygotic) twin pairs. There have been increasing numbers of twin studies with varied approaches, such as those investigating the effects of therapies and their relationship to metabolites, microbiome, epigenetic events, and variability in specific DNA sequences. These comparisons are attractive because of the nearly identical genes evident in monozygotic twins (there are some slight differences such as copy number variations) and the differences evident in fraternal twins. In terms of comparative effectiveness research, the presence of [nearly] identical genes can serve as an opportunity for study, such as:

- **Assessing comparators in individuals with a common genetic profile.** Monozygotic twins may form the comparison pair to test possible treatment options. Unlike the N-of-1 trial in which genetic traits are held constant within the same person, the monozygotic twins control for genetic traits using a parallel trial with two arms (i.e., each member of a twin set assigned to a different treatment arm). There is an advantage of using monozygotic twins instead the N-of-1 approach when the investigator expects that there may be possible carryover effects of the therapies.
- **Evaluating comparators in the context of different genetic-environment influences.** There may also be studies in which both fraternal and monozygotic twins are included. Sometimes such comparisons can help to sort out the effects therapies such as vaccines or to evaluate differences in symptomology (e.g., pain response) with better knowledge of genetic versus environmental influences.
- **Providing information so as to target interventions in individuals with specific characteristics.** There are instances when information from twin or genetic studies can be utilized for planning the design of future comparative effectiveness research studies. Twin studies can provide clues regarding the types of subjects who may be likely candidates for therapies. This can be particularly useful in studies of pharmacogenetics.
- **Providing information to improve the types of interventions offered.** When planning a comparative effectiveness research study, knowing the results of twin studies may inform the investigator regarding the types

of interventions that may potentially show an effect. For example, there was an interesting twin study that did not find a causal relationship between exercise and a reduction in the symptoms of anxiety and depression (DeMoor, 2008), although randomized controlled trials did. It is freely available online if you wish to take a look (http://archpsyc.jamanetwork.com/article.aspx?articleid=210112). The authors were able to tease out the influence of genetic factors that influence voluntary leisure-time exercise. One conclusion was that certain controlled exercise programs (e.g., as a part of a specific monitored therapeutic regimen) could possibly reduce depressive symptoms, while voluntary exercise might be less beneficial in relieving symptoms in patients with depression. This could very well lead to a comparative effectiveness research study in which the types and structures of the regimented exercise programs could be assessed for effect.

Surveys

A survey is an instrument or method of gathering information on people, generally from a sample derived from a larger population. Often surveys are collected in a cross-sectional fashion. That is, at a particular point in time, a questionnaire may be administered to a group of people, who may be defined by region, demographics, or other attributes. Sometimes, if conducted over the Web, the survey may be accessible to many people worldwide.

For purposes of comparative effectiveness research, such surveys may provide information that can be used to extract measures for decision analyses, can be appended to longitudinal retrospective studies, or can be linked with data from time series or panel studies. Before you embark upon your own survey, you should become familiar with large surveys which have been completed and are available for use, or which are currently underway. Some surveys are repeatedly conducted over time so that they may technically constitute a panel study. Others have been conducted only at a specific point in time.

Large population-based surveys are often administered on a national basis in many countries. Such surveys can provide information regarding specific research questions of interest. Critical factors in deciding whether to utilize such information from surveys relate to the following elements:

- **Is the information generalizable to the population of interest?**
  Examine whether the survey captures information from a random sample of households or individuals, or by other methods. Random samples reduce the likelihood of biases based on the types of people chosen for the survey. Other times, representative samples may be taken. That is, the sampling is done to ensure that people in different regions or of different demographic characteristics are adequately

represented. This may be important so that the answers to the questions are a reflection of what occurs in a variety of people.
- **Are the questions used valid and reliable?** There are methods for assessing the accuracy and reproducibility of questions utilized in surveys. Large population-based surveys often include questions that demonstrate rigor in terms of these qualities. At times, there are standardized ways of asking a question and the standards may provide a guide for researchers when assessing health behaviors and health-related conditions.
- **When was the information gathered?** Many health-related practices and behaviors change over time. It is important to know whether the time frame that was captured reflects the period of interest for the comparative effectiveness research question.
- **Is this information potentially linkable to other data?** For some applications in comparative effectiveness, it may be useful to obtain information from multiple sources. The prevalence of certain behaviors, services, or disorders may be extracted from surveys and may be linkable to other databases, for example, by geographical region or by other common elements.

Some databases from national surveys are freely accessible, and files can be downloaded online. Examples of such surveys in the United States are:

- National Health Interview Survey
- National Health and Nutrition Examination Survey
- National Hospital Discharge Survey
- National Health Care Surveys
- National Immunization Survey
- Behavioral Risk Factor Surveillance Survey
- National Vital Statistics System
- National Survey of Family Growth
- Medical Expenditure Panel Survey
- American Community Survey
- American Housing Survey
- National Survey of Children's Health

Take A Look
Look for the American FactFinder (http://factfinder2.census.gov). You can search by geographic region. Go ahead and type in your hometown or a city that is of interest to you within the search box under Community Facts. See what types of demographic information are available. The Census utilizes surveys to acquire information regarding persons in an entire population.

If you are interested in the National Health Interview Survey, the Minnesota Population Center at the University of Minnesota developed an Integrated Health Interview Series (https://www.ihis.us/ihis/). They took data from all the National Health Interview Surveys since the 1960s and linked the variables into a comprehensive system. The integrated system houses individual data and links such personal characteristics across many measures. There is open access for researchers (with registration), and the data are downloadable for use in your

> **Take A Look**
> Go online to the Surveys and Data Collection Systems at the Centers for Disease Control and Prevention (http://www.cdc.gov/nchs/surveys.htm). These surveys are housed within the National Center for Health Statistics. There you will find the links to several public health surveys in the United States. Explore a few of these surveys. For example, within the National Health and Nutrition Examination Survey (NHANES), you will find the questionnaires, datasets, and documentation all online. Many researchers have utilized these datasets. NHANES includes both a physical examination and interviews, and therefore has additional information regarding body measurements and laboratory values that other surveys do not always contain.

> **Take A Look**
> Go to the Aging Integrated Database online (http://www.agidnet.org/). Investigate the types of information available in the maps, charts, and tables. Try to find one area that is of interest to you. Are you able to find information that you did not previously know? Also look at the Data Files section to see the types of data available. Another useful site for geriatrics research is the National Archive of Computerized Data on Aging (http://www.icpsr.umich.edu/icpsrweb/NACDA/). This is the largest library of aging-related electronic data in the United States.

statistical software package. The types of data available for extraction can be tailored, in greater detail, than in many other publicly available databases.

The Aging Integrated Database (http://www.agidnet.org/) combines information from surveys, the census, and other data sources to provide information for research and consumer purposes. Such integrated sites can be useful for locating different types of data on the same population—in this case, geriatrics.

Other sources of health-related data. Although not a survey, the largest database of hospital inpatient information in the United States from all types of payers (i.e., from private insurance, public insurance, and the uninsured) is the Healthcare Cost and Utilization Project (HCUP) which is available for research purposes (http://www.hcup-us.ahrq.gov/). There are several useful databases within this system and below are listed several of the commonly used databases:

- The Nationwide Inpatient Sample, which provides hospital data on adults.
- The Kids' Inpatient Database, which provides hospital data on children.
- The Nationwide Emergency Department Sample contains information on emergency department visits and includes data for both visits that do and do not result in hospital admission.
- The State Ambulatory Surgery Databases, which has same-day surgery data.

There are also individual state-level data at HCUP for hospital and emergency department data, as well as other ancillary files to assist with data management and analyses.

A good central site for health-related data in the United States is HealthData.gov (http://www.healthdata.gov/). Hundreds of databases are listed and are categorized for searching purposes, such as health care providers, epidemiology, children's health, and treatments. Another good central site is the Partners in Information Access for the Public Health Workforce (http://phpartners.org/). Click on their Health Data Tools and Statistics option under Main Topic

Pages to investigate the wide range of data available. You should also check out the Integrated Public Use Microdata Series, which combines census data for research purposes (https://usa.ipums.org/usa/index.shtml). You can select variables by person or household characteristics. There is also an international version, the Integrated Public Use Microdata Series International that includes 68 countries (last count), 211 censuses, and 480 million people! See https://international.ipums.org/international/index.shtml. SodaPop is available as well (http://sodapop.pop.psu.edu/). SodaPop stands for the PennState Online Data Archive for Population Studies. Data downloads are available for many different surveys and health-related databases.

If you are interested in group-level data on health indicators, the Health Indicators Warehouse might be a good source of data to consider (http://healthindicators.gov/). You can link health indicators with evidence-based interventions, and you can chart, graph, and map the data. You may select indicators of interest to you, look at their output by demographics and other health-related measures, and then can download the data in various formats. Visual displays online are also available.

The Health Resources and Services Administration, within the Department of Health and Human Services, houses datasets regarding provider resources. Examples include the National Sample Survey of Registered Nurses, physician characteristics in Primary Care Service Areas, data regarding Health Professional Shortage Areas, and links to the Area Health Resource file. If you visit the data warehouse at this site (http://datawarehouse.hrsa.gov/), you can select the downloadable data of your choice. You may also directly visit the Area Health Resource File site (http://www.arf.hrsa.gov/). It contains a wide variety of information related to the health care professions, training, facilities, expenditures, and the population by county in the United States.

The Inter-University Consortium for Political and Social Research houses more than 70 data files that can be utilized by researchers (http://www.icpsr.umich.edu/icpsrweb/landing.jsp). Many of the public health databases can be found there, as well as databases related to social services, the law, education, and demography. Within Find and Analyze Data, if you select Health Care and Facilities under Browse by Topic, you will see hundreds of results. Data are sometimes available and can be downloaded in a various formats.

If you are interested in data regarding injuries, the Web-Based Injury Statistics Query and Reporting System (WISQARS) will allow you to extract both fatal and nonfatal injury data, as well as violent deaths (http://www.cdc.gov/injury/wisqars/index.html). Years of potential life lost, types of injuries, costs, demographics, and geographic data are available. CDC Wonder is another query site for public health data (http://wonder.cdc.gov/). This site allows access to several public health databases. Click on the Topics tab on the top and see the types of information available.

The National Quality Measures Clearinghouse is a useful site for those researchers who intend to include within their study evidence-based quality measures and various measure sets that are used in research and practice (http://www.qualitymeasures.ahrq.gov/). This site does not contain survey-level data on patients, but if you are utilizing quality measures as primary or secondary outcomes, you might look at the types of measures used. These are generally group-level outcomes such as "percentage of patients with low back pain diagnosis who are prescribed opioids" or "percent of pediatric asthma inpatients who received relievers during hospitalization."

If you are studying nutrition, keep in mind that there are databases available from the US Department of Agriculture regarding the Supplemental Nutrition Assistance Program, Food Distribution Programs, School Meals, and Women, Infants, and Children program. USDA also houses databases regarding food safety and food consumption. Databases are downloadable onsite.

The US Department of Energy houses a series of health-related databases at the Comprehensive Epidemiologic Data Resource site that are available for downloading (https://www3.orau.gov/CEDR/default.aspx#.UewZA21hSVI). The National Institute for Occupational Safety and Health houses an Emergency Response Safety and Health Database that is worth checking out (http://www.cdc.gov/niosh/ershdb/) if you wish to obtain data regarding emergencies and disasters.

If you are studying a specific disease or population, you might want to check out the specific National Health Institute associated with the condition or population (e.g., macular degeneration at the National Eye Institute). Each Institute funds different population-relevant research and links to their studies and databases may be available.

The European Health for All Database is located at the World Health Organization (Regional Europe Office) and contains data regarding health status, determinants, risk factors, resources, and utilization for 53 countries (last count). It is available to use online or to download. The Council of European Social Science Data Archives is an organization that provides access to over 25,000 data collections for research use (http://www.cessda.org/). If you select the CESSDA Catalogue under Accessing Data, you can search by keywords. Many topics are available such as accidents and injuries, childbearing, drug use, general health, health care, health policy, nutrition, physical fitness, and specific diseases. Try typing in "statins" and see what results are retrieved.

If you are conducting international research, the Global Health Observatory of the World Health Organization contains data on mortality, disease burden, child and maternal health, immunizations, infectious and noninfectious diseases, environmental factors, violence and injuries, health systems, and other measures (http://www.who.int/gho/en/). The World Bank also has a section regarding data pertaining to health, nutrition, and population data (http://data.worldbank.org/). There are also International Human Development Indicators (http://hdr.undp.org/en/statistics/) and Millennium Development Goals Indicators (http://mdgs.un.org/unsd/mdg/Default.aspx) listed at the United Nations site. Data can be downloaded or displayed onsite (try out the Public Data Explorer).

The Global Health Data Exchange at the University of Washington contains demographic and health data for many countries throughout the world (http://ghdx.healthmetricsandevaluation.org/). The International Household Survey Network is another central site for obtaining data (http://www.ihsn.org/home/). Datasets, when available, are listed and are accessible after registration. The original questionnaire can also be downloaded as a pdf.

While you are exploring these databases, you may notice that some sites have specific tools available such as mechanisms for data extraction. DataFerrett is one such tool (http://dataferrett.census.gov/) and stands for Federated Electronic Research, Review, Extraction, and Tabulation Tool. It will allow you to retrieve data from several large surveys, such as the National Hospital Ambulatory Medical Care Survey and the National Health Interview Survey. You can generate tables via several different formats and then import these into your statistical package.

Systematic Reviews and Meta-Analysis

Decision making regarding possible therapeutic choices is often enhanced by an evaluation of the evidence across many studies, all meant to address a single research question. What if you locate six trials and they all suggest a somewhat similar effect, but there is some lingering doubt about the true effect? There are ways in which such evidence can be reviewed and combined across studies. Such studies are particularly informative when they are inclusive of all evidence on a particular topic. That is, one would prefer to not selectively accept the results of just some studies, and throw out the others. Rather, one would make an attempt to review all the evidence in a meaningful fashion. There are two main types of integrative approaches that are frequently used:

- **Systematic reviews** are investigations in which evidence is assembled regarding a particular research question across all original research studies that meet specific preset criteria.
- **A meta-analysis** is a study in which the results of systematic reviews are mathematically combined.

The common method for gathering original research studies is to locate databases that serve as repositories for such studies. The Medical Literature Analysis and Retrieval System online (MEDLINE) is one of the databases that contains journal citations and bibliographic data related to publications in medicine, dentistry, nursing, pharmacology, and other health disciplines. Citations on original research articles are housed, dating from the 1940s, in this database founded by the National Library of Medicine in the United States. Searching for articles is freely available online through PubMed. Embase is another database frequently used for systematic reviews. It is a global repository of published biomedical research articles and has extensive coverage. It is particularly good in the retrieval of drug information beyond that captured for life science articles in general. The Cochrane Central Register of Controlled Trials (CENTRAL) is another source, as are other trial registries (e.g., http://www.clinicaltrials.gov; http://apps.who.int/trialsearch/). The Cumulative Index to Nursing and Allied Health Literature (CINAHL) and PsycINFO are additional sources used to retrieve citations of original research studies, as are Scopus and the Web of Science. Depending upon the research topic of interest, there may also be national or regional biolographic databases or subject-specific databases which can be searched. Citation indices such as Scopus or the Web of Science may also be used. For those investigators interested in searching conference proceedings for abstracts, Open Grey (http://www.opengrey.eu/) allows open access for searching the grey literature (dissertations, reports, abstracts from conferences). ProQuest (http://www.proquest.co.uk/en-UK/catalogs/databases/detail/pqdt.shtml) provides searching dissertations and theses for a fee and the National Technical Information Services provides open-access searching for technical reports (http://www.ntis.gov/). Previous published reviews may be a source for locating original research although it should not be the sole source. Occasionally, handsearching of journals may be conducted in specific instances.

Discover

Search for the Cochrane Handbook for Systematic Reviews of Interventions online (http://handbook.cochrane.org/). Look at the information available in each chapter. Also go to the Institute of Medicine site online. Search for Standards for Systematic Reviews of Comparative Effectiveness Research (http://iom.edu/Reports/2011/Finding-What-Works-in-Health-Care-Standards-for-Systematic-Reviews.aspx). You can download their pdf book for no charge. If you plan to conduct your own systematic review and meta-analysis in the future, keep these sources in mind.

Conducting a systematic review and meta-analysis is a structured process. Gold standards for this process were developed by the Cochrane collaboration, a global network of professionals dedicated to using high-quality timely research evidence to advance decision making in health care. The group is named after Dr. Archie (Archibald) Cochrane, a British epidemiologist, who sought to use systematic and scientific evidence to answer questions regarding treatment and medical care. Take a look at the website for the Cochrane Collaboration (www.cochrane.org). If you do follow this line of research and conduct systematic reviews with a research team in the future, you will no doubt benefit from reading through their Cochrane Handbook, which is online.

The process of systematic review and meta-analysis is well defined. However, to illustrate the general procedures and to condense it into some basic steps, the process generally follows this reasoning:

1. **Define the research question or hypothesis.** This would follow the template previously described by the acronym PICOTS: Patient, Intervention, Comparison, Outcome, Timing, and Setting. The investigators would decide the eligibility criteria for study inclusion. Questions such as "Do we include studies that used patients of all ages, or do we restrict the review to adults only?" should be addressed. There may be additional selection criteria based on the type of interventions of interest. For comparative effectiveness research, we would be reviewing studies in which one viable therapy would be compared with another or several alternate therapies. The definitions for all comparators need to be clarified and outcomes of interest should be prespecified. Timing is another consideration—both in terms of capturing studies by years in which they were published and also by consideration of the lengths of follow-up minimally required for the studies to be included (when applicable to the research question). Setting may also define the research question. For example, some reviews are conducted for patients in critical care settings only while others may be restricted to studies conducted in emergency department settings and so forth.
2. **Draft the protocol that you will use for your review process.** Include the research question and the decision made regarding patients, intervention, comparison, and outcomes as listed above. As you step through the following procedures, add these items to your protocol. Use established guidelines that have been developed for systematic reviews and meta-analysis as guides through this process (http://www.equator-network.org).
3. **Decide on the bibliographic databases that you will use to search for articles.** Make a list of all the sources that will be searched. Often, the Cochrane Central Register of Controlled Trials, MEDLINE and Embase are used for searching. You may want to consider consulting with an experienced reference librarian regarding your options. Also determine the dates of the studies that you would like included. This may be from the inception of the publication database to the current date. Specify the language of the studies. Ideally, one would prefer to include all studies, regardless of language, and articles could be translated if necessary.
4. **Develop the search terms to use for each electronic database.** Here again, it may be helpful to work with a medical librarian who has experience with the types of search terms utilized in the databases.

There may be differences in the search strings, based on the particular bibliographic database. For example, MEDLINE uses MeSH or Medical Subject Headings (http://www.nlm.nih.gov/mesh/meshhome.html).

5. **Conduct the search within each database as specified in your protocol.** In addition, keep a record of the search results throughout the searching process. For example, record the number of articles retrieved within each database (e.g., 1279 articles in MEDLINE, 1455 articles in Embase, etc.).
6. **Examine the abstracts to determine whether each one meets your inclusion criteria.** Generally this is done by two independent reviewers (i.e., reviewers are blinded or masked to each other's assignments). Record the number of abstracts that do not meet the criteria and keep a record of the reason why they did not meet these criteria (incorrect population, not a randomized controlled trial, did not assess your specific intervention of interest, etc.).
7. **When the abstract review is completed by both reviewers, assign a third and experienced unbiased researcher to assess agreement and disagreement and to serve as an adjudicator.** Resolve any disagreements through discussion with the adjudicator and through final vote by the three researchers. Record the number of disagreements and reasons. Kappa statistics or other measures of concordance can be calculated.
8. **Pull the original full-length research articles that fit the inclusion criteria.** Include the entire article as well as supplemental data, tables, and figures.
9. **Develop an abstraction form to extract information from each eligible research study.** This often includes names of authors, year of publication, and location of the study; types of patients or participants, the number of participants enrolled in the study, and the number of participants who completed the study; demographic characteristics of the participants; details regarding the types of therapies or interventions assessed in each arm; description of the outcomes; other relevant information that you would consider important to this particular hypothesis; and extract numbers relevant to the results. These would include the numbers of people in each arm of the study, the numbers of people who experienced the outcome, and other statistics relevant to calculating the results, if a meta-analysis is planned.
10. **Describe all the eligible studies that are included in the systematic review.** Provide a summary of the descriptive elements of each study in a table, which will be included in the final publication (often this is Table 1). Such descriptive information includes subject characteristics, where the study was performed, the study design, elements relevant to the intervention, the number of subjects, and other relevant data.

11. **Examine each study for the possibility of bias (systematic error).** The features of each study that relate to bias or avoidance of bias should be noted. For example, concealed randomization helps to prevent selection bias. Blinding of outcome assessment abates detection bias. The degree of incomplete follow-up or attrition rates should be recorded. Whether the analyses were conducted as intent-to-treat should also be reported. The Cochrane Collaboration has a domain-based evaluation for bias which is particularly helpful to prepare if the review contains solely randomized trials. When meta-analyses are conducted, the investigator may stratify the results based on the presence or absence of particular biases.

12. **Describe the results in the studies.** What were the principal findings from the studies? Often the results comparing two therapies are expressed as ratios: odds ratios, relative risks, risk ratios, or hazard ratios. Sometimes the results comparing two therapies are given as risk differences (that is, the risks are subtracted instead of divided). Occasionally, the results are in the form of absolute proportions or rates. It is also possible to see results presented with different types of measures than the usual epidemiologic measures stated above (e.g., in some social science research, mean differences or correlation coefficients may be used in the original research studies).

13. **Calculate a summary or pooled measure if the studies do not show appreciable heterogeneity.** There are different methods for pooling depending upon the type of statistic being pooled (or summarized). In a fixed model, the variance within each study is utilized to calculate summary values. In a random model, both the variance within each study and the variance between studies are used to calculate summary values. Statistical packages are available for meta-analyses and other procedures associated with this analysis. It is critical that the correct information is extracted from each article for each of these measures and, if additional calculations are necessary to obtain a common statistic across all articles, it is important that the calculations are correct. Statistics regarding heterogeneity should be included and often sensitivity analyses are performed. If heterogeneity exists, reasons for such heterogeneity are often explored. There are statistical techniques for evaluating publication bias, as well as for influential studies and other contributing factors. Sometimes meta-regression is performed.

14. **Prepare the tables and figures showing the results, quality of the studies, and a summary of the findings.** Start drafting your methods and results sections for publication. Prepare the forest plots for presentation. If you are new to this process, take a look at some meta-analyses in the published literature

> **Explore**
>
> You can begin to see the elements required for a systematic review and meta-analysis by looking at published examples. First go to the medical literature (e.g., search for PubMed). Search for "meta-analysis." Look at some of the meta-analyses reported in the major medical journals (*Annals of Internal Medicine* contain some good examples). Look at their structure. Generally, they appear a bit longer than an original research article in journals. What usually is presented in Table 1? What types of information do you see in the other tables? Now check their figures. See any figures that show forest plots? See how these forest plots look and how they vary from one article to another. Check any other types of graphs that you see in these publications. Look at several meta-analyses in major medical journals. Do you see a general pattern of the types of information presented?

15. **Interpret your results and place them in context of real-world settings.** State your conclusions and recommendations. Finish writing the complete manuscript and review among all the authors. Now you are ready to submit your manuscript to a journal for publication.

Relevant Features of Meta-Analysis: There are several distinct features in meta-analysis, such as:

- **Forest Plots.** These types of plots visually summarize the results from the individual studies as well as display the pooled (or summary) estimate. An example is given in Figure 5.7. The exact appearance may vary somewhat, but generally, the first author and year of publication are given on the left-hand side. In the middle are the results of the studies with point estimates and 95% confidence intervals. Sometimes the sample size for each study and the weights used for pooling are given as well. At times the forest plot can be simple, giving the results comparing one therapy to another (often with relative risks or odds ratios) for a specific outcome. Other times the forest plot can be more complicated, with multiple outcomes shown and stratification by particular study characteristics. It has been said that a picture is worth a thousand words; the forest plot is a clear gem in terms of showing the results in a manner that most readers can understand.

- **Cumulative meta-analysis.** There are instances in which the studies in a meta-analysis are first sorted by year of publication, starting with the oldest first and finishing with the most recent study. When this is done, the results of the oldest study are given at the top of the forest plot. As each sequential study is listed (by publication year), its findings are combined with the previous results. The second line on the forest plot uses the data from the first and second studies. The third line on the forest plot uses the data from the first, second, and third studies. This continues until the end of the plot. Therefore, as each study is published, the summary values are pooled. At the bottom of the forest plot is the summary (pooled) value for all studies. The forest plot for a cumulative meta-analysis (Figure 5.8)

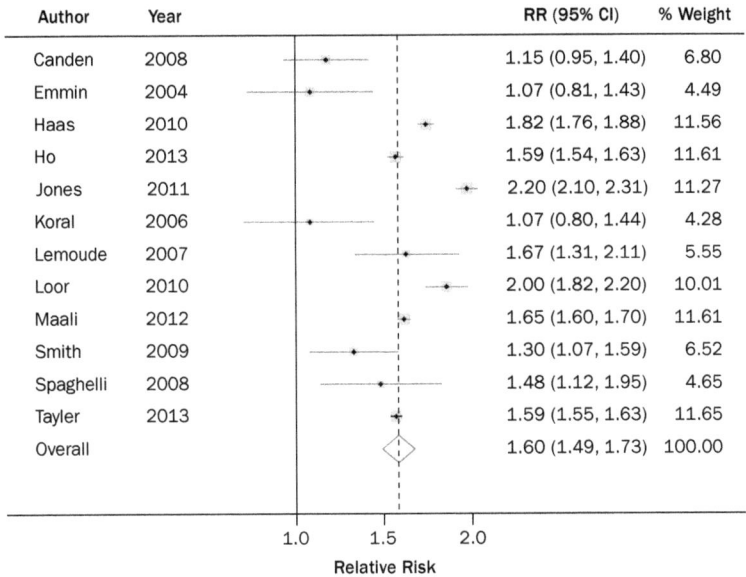

FIGURE 5.7 Example of a Forest Plot.

has a distinctly different look than the forest plot for a regular meta-analysis, in which all studies are pooled together at the end. The final summary estimate will actually be the same for each of these two methods (cumulative and regular), but the look of the forest plots will be different. A cumulative forest plot can give you a clue as to whether there were likely consistent treatment effects through calendar time. Sometimes publication of cumulative forest plots can help researchers

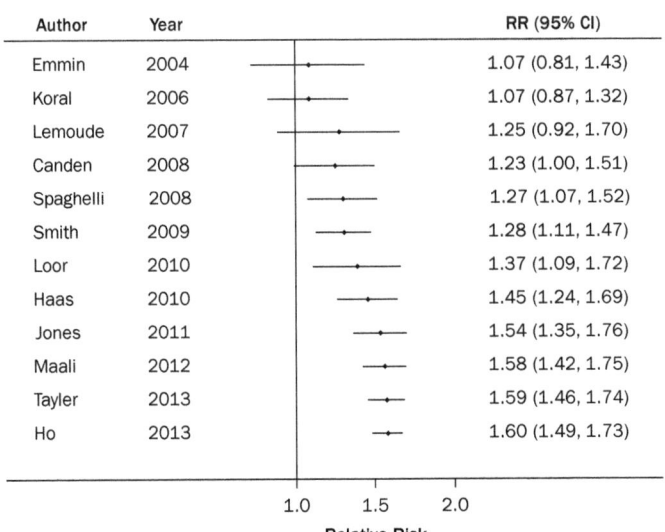

FIGURE 5.8 Example of a Forest Plot with Cumulative Meta-Analysis.

see temporal patterns in the evidence. The underlying reasons for these patterns are generally investigated.
- **Influence assessment in meta-analysis.** Influence analysis is a way of checking for outliers. That is, there may be a specific study that, when removed from the meta-analysis, causes the remaining results to change. When this study is removed, the results shift. Such a study can be influential in interpreting the results.
- **Heterogeneity in meta-analysis.** Heterogeneity refers to between-study differences in the results. Sometimes the difference in effect among the various studies is so great that the results cannot be pooled. There are various statistical measures used to assess heterogeneity. When you conduct your first meta-analysis, you'll learn more details about each of these measures.
- **Proteus effect in meta-analysis.** This is when the first study ever conducted on the topic shows an extreme result but all the following studies do not. It suggests that the first study may have been published because of an unusual finding, but upon further examination in other studies, the true effect (or lack thereof) becomes more evident.

Decision Modeling

Decision modeling is an umbrella term used to describe a variety of procedures which use existing data and underlying assumptions regarding the behavior of events in the real world to generate mathematical models so to inform decision making. These approaches use mathematics or statistics, but often in different ways. The researcher can investigate which decisions lead to better outcomes in patients, the timing of the decisions, and how these relate to outcomes, as well as the degree of uncertainly and the impact of additional information. Often, such procedures integrate data from demographic, epidemiologic, economic, social, clinical, and other health-related sources. It is not uncommon for decision modeling studies to utilize an interdisciplinary approach with scientists from different fields of study.

In some ways, decision modeling is akin to meta-analysis in that the researcher is integrating evidence from multiple sources. Decision modeling is a rapidly evolving area in comparative effectiveness research which is facilitated by the availability of linked electronic databases containing information that is relevant to treatment choices, and containing longitudinal data regarding outcomes in large populations.

There are several common decision models used in health research:
- **Decision trees.** These methods utilize information regarding the probability of events and their consequences to inform decisions.

Generally, graphical models or algorithms are displayed showing the decisions of relevance to the topic of interest, the set of outcomes and their probabilities after a decision is made, and a final endpoint indicating value or worth to an individual. Decisions can be simulated based on the value of the outcome status to the patient, taking into account the probabilities of occurrences in the causal pathway.

- **Markov models.** In these methods, a cohort of people can be simulated over time as they transition to different health states. Markov models can be utilized within the context of decision trees to better simulate the natural progression of disease over time. Options are available, such as fixed state transition probabilities (Markov chains) or time-dependent transition probabilities (Markov processes). Time-dependent transition probabilities are often utilized when modeling chronic disease (as people age) over longer periods of time.
- **Monte Carlo simulation.** In these iterative models, events in people are modeled over time with their state transitions and outcomes simulated by sampling either known or estimated distributions. An example is the MIcrosimulation for Screening Analysis (MISCAN), used to simulate both cancer progression and screening. Search for this online and you will see examples of how these models are used to predict outcomes with various types of cancer screening protocols (e.g., http://www.ncbi.nlm.nih.gov/books/NBK34018/).
- **Discrete event simulation.** These are methods whereby sequences of events are modeled over time to assess the effect on systems. Timing of the events is precisely defined, as are the types of event changes. It is a dynamic model that changes over time and is often used for the prediction of complex events. For example, in some cancer applications, information is utilized regarding polyp incidence rates at specific ages as well as the size and growth rate of the polyps.
- **Microsimulation.** These are methods usually conducted to predict future risk whereby events are modeled in individuals or groups by their attributes. Often many different sources of data are utilized to inform the model. An example is Health Forecasting (http://www.health-forecasting.org/), developed by researchers in the UCLA Fielding School of Public Health. Check out their Health Forecasting Toolkit, in which you can create a quick report online using their model or can login for more advanced features. Another example is the Population Health Model (POHEM), which was developed by Canadian researchers to simulate life trajectories for the population based on information regarding sociodemographic factors, health behaviors, disease incidence, costs, and mortality (http://www.phac-aspc.gc.ca/ph-sp/php-psp/php3-eng.php#Developing).

> **Check It Out**
> You may get a sense of the output from various models by looking at their images. Go online and search for "decision tree" in Images. Scroll down and look at the output associated with various decision trees. Do you see some favorites? Now type in "Markov model" or "Markov chain" in Images and scroll down to see the images. Also type in "discrete event simulation" and look at the graphics. Lastly, type in "dynamic model" to see what types of images come up. Find anything interesting?

- **Dynamic models.** These methods incorporate change, feedback loops, and complex states through sets of differential and algebraic equations to simulate alterations in health and interactions over time. An example is a model called ReThink Health (and its earlier version, HealthBound), which is a dynamic model built to simulate and test assumptions regarding large-scale interventions such as delivering care, expanding health insurance coverage, encouraging healthier behavior, and improving environmental conditions (http://rippelfoundation.org/rethink-health/dynamics/). The researchers found that encouraging healthier behavior and improving environmental conditions (historically labeled "primary prevention" in public health and preventive medicine) yielded better long-term health outcomes with cost savings. You can try it out online at the Fannie E. Rippel Foundation site (http://rippelfoundation.org/rethink-health/dynamics/local-rethink-health-models/).

Sometimes it is easier to imagine these models and their objectives by looking at some examples. One example is the decision that adults make regarding colorectal cancer screening. Possible choices include colonoscopy, flexible sigmoidoscopy, and fecal occult blood tests. To assist individuals regarding which test to use and when, researchers used microsimulation models to estimate how many years of life one would gain by using these three screening tests.

> **Search**
> Search online for the *Annals of Internal Medicine*. Click on the Advanced Search Option. For the Citation search, type in Year 2008, Volume 149, and First Page 659. This should lead you to an article called "Evaluating Test Strategies for Colorectal Cancer Screening: A Decision Analysis for the US Preventive Services Task Force." Read through the article. Look over the types of information collected and the way the results are given. Using these two microsimulation models, at what age should someone start screening? Which tests were associated with the longer number of life-years gained?

In this chapter, many of the more common designs are described. Because the types of interventions and outcomes in comparative effectiveness research are diverse, there may be other options and variations. Feel free to search for other designs when your research question does not quite fit into any of the designs listed here.

6

The Person

Go to a quiet place. Sit down and think. What makes you who you are? How would you describe yourself as a person? Would you begin with a description of your physical characteristics—that is, how you look to other people? Would you define yourself in terms of your temperament or your demeanor? Would you describe yourself in terms of how you react with other people? Are you defined by your thoughts, dreams, and aspirations?

A bit of introspection regarding who you are as a person helps to understand the complexities of describing individuals. Some people write blogs, diaries, or journals listing their activities and thoughts. Some chronicle their lives in a book: Who they were as a child, how their development changed their perspectives, and how events in their lives shaped what they achieved. You could probably fill volumes with descriptive elements of your experiences.

Some of this introspection provides opportunities to realize certain underlying commonalities. There are similarities in the types of events that occur in people—especially when you start to think about those factors that often drive these events. There may be similar health-related behaviors and disorders that occur throughout our lifespans, from infancy through childhood and as adults. Often, in health research, we try to capture such common characteristics and group people by these factors. You may fit into the 30- to 39-year-old male category with no previous history of hypertension or diabetes mellitus – or maybe not.

But for all the categorizations that we attempt, there is the underlying realization that we are all unique. Even identical twins raised in the same household are not exactly the same. There are different interactions and exposures throughout their lifetimes. Some of this attention to our uniqueness is reflected in an area of research and practice called personalized medicine. This greater personalization of health care is an important aspect of comparative effectiveness research. One of the objectives is to answer the question, "What works best for me?"

Precision Medicine and Personalized Medicine

Precision medicine and personalized medicine are closely related areas in which therapies and services are more finely tailored to the specific attributes of the individual. Often, it has come to indicate consideration of both the genetic make-up of a person (genotype) and the observable traits (phenotype) in the larger context of their social and physical environment. Being able to tailor treatments and services to the unique attributes of an individual is appealing, because we know that both genotype and phenotype are associated with disease risk. Specific gene mutations have been shown to be associated with cancers, sickle cell disease, cystic fibrosis, Alzheimer's disease, cardiovascular disease, and many other conditions. If you searched the literature in depth, you might be hard-pressed to find a disease that doesn't have some genetic aspect. Risk stratification by observable traits such as smoking status, body mass index, and other health-related factors has been conducted within research studies for some time. Now we have additional availabilities of genetic data and, at times, the possibility of greater access to real-time phenotypic data to fine-tune such approaches.

There are subtle differences regarding the use of the terms precision medicine and personalized medicine. Precision medicine has more to do with using additional information to better understand the types of diseases and disorders that a person has in order to maximize potential benefit from certain therapies while minimizing adverse effects. If a child has a developmental disorder that affects her cognition, greater knowledge of this particular disorder and how it affects this child may open opportunities for more targeted therapies. Personalized medicine, while sometimes used in this context, was initially utilized to indicate the application of genetic information to pharmacologic data in order to fine-tune the types of therapies in which a particular patient would respond. Some of the interest spawned from drug trials in which the same chemical compound was having differing effects in people—a phenomenon sometimes called the heterogeneity of treatment effect. However, in humans many traits are multigenic and, even if one knows the genes of a patient, there are sometimes differences in gene expression and alternative splicing that cannot be discerned by just knowing the alleles of a gene. Humans turned out to be a bit more complex than at first glance. Moreover, some practitioners had second thoughts about the term "personalized" because, in ordinary practice, of course one tries to personalize therapies to patients on a daily basis. In any case, sometimes you will find that personalized medicine and precision medicine are used interchangeably in the medical literature while, at other times, people make these distinctions.

Discover

Go to the National Academy of Sciences site and look at a report called "Toward Precision Medicine: Building a Knowledge Network for Biomedical Research and a New Taxonomy of Disease." You can download a copy of the report (the pdf is free). The summary or brief is available here (http://dels.nas.edu/resources/static-assets/materials-based-on-reports/reports-in-brief/precision-med-final.pdf). Check out the illustration regarding how the data layers in precision medicine parallel the layering approach by geographic information systems. When you scan through the summary, are all the terms familiar? What is the exposome?

Greater examination of the heterogeneity of treatment effect is a response to many of the questions that patients often ask. Why do some therapies seem to work in most people but don't work in others? Why do some individuals have no or few adverse effects from a given medication while others develop serious complications? Such questions are very important, and form the basis of a discipline called pharmacogenetics. In pharmacogenetic studies, DNA samples may be obtained from participants (sometimes from a buccal swab or a blood draw). After this sample is analyzed, the genetic information is combined with other clinical information from patients regarding their use of various medications, their medical history, and their personal characteristics. Large databases of such information hold the potential for providing valuable in identifying which types of people are at greater risk of adverse effects and which are most likely to beneficially respond to treatment. When such studies are complete, this information can be used to update drug labels with data regarding response variability to genomic biomarkers, risk for adverse events, and genotype-specific dosing.

Applications of precision medicine have been explored in cancer research with the discovery of several protein receptors that affect prognosis. For example, expression of human epidermal growth factor receptor 2 (HER2) is known to be related to breast cancer recurrence and is utilized in drugs that bind specifically to these receptors. Individuals can be tested for the presence of HER2 and this can inform therapeutic options.

> **Tip**
> It is not uncommon to hear the words "genetic" and "inherited" in the lay press, especially when discussing cancer. From a scientific point of view, keep in mind the difference between these terms. Mutations that occur in gamete cells (think egg and sperm) can be passed on to the next generation and therefore, are heritable. However, mutations that occur in somatic cells are not inherited. The words "inherited" and "genetic" are different. All cancers are genetic in origin—that is, they are caused by DNA mutations. Some of these mutations may occur in somatic cells and some mutations occur in germ line cells. Only the mutations present in gametes are heritable. For many cancers, however, it is the combination of different mutations which are the likely culprits.

Precision and personalized medicine also have applications in comparative effectiveness research. If the study design is an N-of-1 trial, the study itself could inform a specific individual of the effectiveness of a therapy. At the end of the N-of-1 trial when all the results are tallied, that person will know which treatment yielded a better effect. Another application in comparative effectiveness research is to structure a study such that predictions would be made regarding the benefits of particular therapies in specific types of people. Usually these are defined by phenotypic groupings, but if genotype information is available, this could be utilized as well. Applications also include systematic reviews and meta-analyses, so that if differences are found in specific types of individuals, these can be recognized. At times, this is done by further examination of heterogeneous effects, either through subgroup analyses or by meta-regression. When research studies employ the use of large electronic databases with deep and diverse data regarding health-related characteristics, there is a greater potential that both beneficial and adverse effects could be identified so that recommendations could be tailored more at the subgroup level.

Describing Participants in a Study

When you read clinical research studies published in the medical literature, one of the first items addressed in the results section is a description of who was in the study. What were the characteristics of the subjects who participated? Often a table is given showing their age, gender, history of medical conditions, and various other factors relevant to the particular investigation. Therefore a researcher can anticipate that, when planning and implementing a study, the collection of this information is necessary. It is critical to the understanding of who responds to specific therapies and who does not. It is critical to interpretation of the results and in recognizing in whom these findings may apply. When you read an article regarding several approaches to the management of inguinal hernia, one of the first items to notice is whether these approaches were conducted in men, women, or children. If you are interested in surgical techniques in pediatric applications, one can easily tease out those investigations that are and are not likely to apply.

Take A Look

Go to PubMed Central (http://www.ncbi.nlm.nih.gov/pmc/) where you will find open access full-text research articles. That is, you will be able to read the entire article online. Type in "pragmatic randomized controlled trial" and look at some of the studies that are retrieved. Select one of the trials and scroll down to see how the investigators described the study population or participants. Sometimes there is a separate section for this description and, at other times, it is incorporated within the methods and results sections. What types of information did they include? Do this for several trials. Are you getting a general idea of different ways in which this information can be incorporated?

Suppose you are designing your own study. Decisions regarding participants in the study are most critical in several areas: (a) deciding who will be eligible to participate in the investigation, (b) deciding which variables to use to describe the subjects once they reach eligibility, and (c) deciding how to use these personal characteristics within the analyses to better clarify the results under investigation. In comparative effectiveness research, there is an attempt to widen eligibility so that all patients who are likely candidates for specific therapies would be included. When the study is complete, it is important to describe the results in sufficient detail so to provide meaningful information regarding the effectiveness of the therapies in subgroups when there is variability in the effect across different types of people.

At the start of a study, once eligibility criteria are defined, which subject-level characteristics should you collect? This is directed by the research questions and hypotheses to be tested. A good starting point for the determination of personal characteristics is to review those factors that are either commonly or strongly related to the outcomes in the study. Perhaps these factors are already known to the investigators but, to ensure that some are not missed, go to the medical literature and search for risk factors for the outcomes and make a fairly comprehensive list. You may also consider asking your colleagues and other experts who deal with the outcome in daily life. For example, if your study involves assessing recovery times (outcome) after a specific surgery, ask your colleagues—the physicians and nurses who take care of patients postoperatively. What patient characteristics affect recovery times? Add the expert-advice types of factors to your list of risk factors you found from the search of the literature.

While at first this process may seem somewhat labor intensive, it is often worth the effort. It is important that factors that are strongly related to the outcomes are considered in the design and implementation of studies. Imagine that you are working with a network of primary care clinics and have access to patient-level information in a large electronic database. You are part of a team that is exploring whether two specific educational approaches affect adherence to medication regimens in persons with type 2 diabetes. You compare adherence rates in both intervention groups (i.e., the two specific educational approaches) and ensure that the subjects are comparable on baseline characteristics by matching on many different factors. Sometimes this matching is done by a method called propensity score matching. At the end of the study, the results are being prepared in a draft of the manuscript for publication. You present the findings at a scientific conference and, afterwards, you are approached by another scientist who asks, "Did you match on literacy?" Oops. Of course, literacy could possibly be related to these educational approaches and may also affect adherence but, somehow this factor was missed during the analysis. This person-level characteristic—the ability to read and write—may be an important factor to consider. Therefore, the database is revisited and this factor is further explored. Going to the extra effort of finding all likely influences on the outcomes during the study design phase can be valuable.

Explore

Go to PubMed Central (http://www.ncbi.nlm.nih.gov/pmc/) and search for "propensity score" and scroll through the types of articles that utilize various propensity score techniques. Are there any investigations that are relevant to comparative effectiveness research?

Keep in mind that patient characteristics most important to evaluate during the design phase involve those items that are (1) strongly related to the outcome; (2) related to both the outcome and the interventions; (3) necessary to form patient-specific subgroups of interest in the data analyses; and (4) necessary to describe the participants to the general public and other health professionals.

Once the list of patient characteristics is formed, then the investigators determine how each of these items will be assessed. One might think that after the list is formed, you just ask each subject this information and be done with it. But there is actually a science underlying how best to collect and record patient-level information in research studies. In electronic databases, often these decisions have already been made and the investigator must use the information as it currently exists. However, if you are a part of a team that inputs data for electronic capture, or you are a part of a prospective study where this information is necessary to collect, there are often standard methods for collecting and reporting variables in scientific studies.

Age: Take something as basic as age. For many studies, just asking someone's age is sufficient. Age at a given time point (e.g., hospital admission) may be adequate for the purposes of a particular study. But current age is relevant in terms of the present calendar time and, for longitudinal studies, this can present a challenge. Age changes with time. If the data are available in a longitudinal database over a 20-year period, there is no single age for each patient. Knowing one's birthdate can provide valuable information so that time between certain events that happen during the subject's life can be calculated, if the dates of the events were included in the study or database. From an analysis point of view, calendar dates for therapies, procedures, and use of specific medical services can be important. With the addition of birthdate, the age of the patient when each of these events occurred can be calculated or the time period between events can be determined.

Beyond the reporting of age in a particular study, there are instances in which aging or lifespan are an integral part of the research question. Especially when researchers have access to longitudinal databases, measures such as longevity, healthy life years, and disability-free life years may be important. The age and date when individuals enter the cohort and the length of time under observation can be critical elements of the research.

Sex: Sex is another baseline personal characteristic generally recorded in studies. Research studies often show the distribution of subjects by listing the percentage of men and women, while other studies restrict enrollment to one sex by virtue of the hypothesis under investigation. In humans, sexual differences originate with genetics. These gene differences are manifested by anatomical variations in structure and stature, as well as by physiologic variations in function (e.g. hormonal differences). Gender, however, refers to the cultural and societal manifestation of such sex differences. From a research point of view, investigators often use the term "sex" when referring to biologic differences and "gender" when referring to the manifestation of such differences in everyday life or society as a whole.

When conducting comparative effectiveness research that is relevant to both genders, plan to include enough participants so that you can present the results separately for males and females. There are many known differences in health-related outcomes by gender and, therefore, it is important that patients know whether there are differing effects in men and women. There are many diseases that show predominance in men and many others that occur more frequently in women. Moreover, there are rich social and cultural aspects of gender that vary with therapies and services, so that this factor may exhibit critical influences on the variables of interest in a study.

Discover

Find ten diseases that are more common in women and ten that are more common in men. Beyond gender differences in disease, try to find gender differences in the use of therapies, medical services, health behaviors, or other factors that may influence health outcomes. Can you name ten of these in women and ten in men?

Race and ethnicity: Race and ethnicity are other personal characteristics that are often included in research studies. Both constructs may have considerable influence on the outcomes of a study and may also relate to health services received. For purposes of many research studies in the United States, a common classification of race is as follows:

- American Indian or Alaska Native (defined as a person having origins in any of the peoples of North and South America, including Central America, and who maintains tribal affiliation or community attachment).
- Asian (defined as a person having origins in any of the peoples of the Far East, Southeast Asia, or the Indian subcontinent, including people from Cambodia, China, India, Japan, Korea, Malaysia, Pakistan, the Philippine Islands, Thailand, and Vietnam).
- Black or African (defined as a person having origins in any of the black racial groups of Africa).
- Native Hawaiian or Other Pacific Islander (defined as a person having origins in any of the peoples of Hawaii, Guam, Samoa, or other Pacific Islands).
- White (defined as a person having origins in any of the peoples of Europe, the Middle East, or North Africa).

With globalization and increasing migration, the use of such categories may be undergoing some reconsideration but in research studies, differences in health outcomes by race are often evident. From a scientific point of view, molecular biologists have provided some perspectives on such groupings. Since all peoples first resided in Africa, Africans have the greatest diversity in genotypes. Asians (who migrated from Africa) and Whites (who also migrated from Africa) have genotypes that were derived from peoples in Africa. Therefore, the genetic diversity seen in Asians and in Whites is less than in Africans. Native Hawaiians, Pacific Islanders, Alaska Natives, and Native Americans are descendants of peoples in Asia, and their genotypes were derived from (and have less diversity than) the Asian population. In some research studies, it may be useful to keep this information in mind; race (using the five categories listed above) does not necessarily group people of differing genetic profiles. The genetic characteristics of Africans will overlap that of Whites and Asians. From purely a scientific perspective, these racial categories do not clearly differentiate genotypes.

So if race (by these five categories) is not mutually exclusive in differentiating genotype, what exactly is this race variable which is usually reported in many research studies? What are we differentiating? This categorization for race seen in the medical literature is basically a historical construct based on phenotype and social and political factors. In current society, it is a factor that differentiates groups of people based on social, behavioral, and environmental elements—all of which impact health.

In many clinical studies, race is defined by the individual being described. It is the person's assessment of his or her own personal and group identity. In practice, however, race may be defined by a number of different people other than the person being described. For example, sometimes it is the coroner who records the race of the person who died. Sometimes it is a parent or an attending physician who describes the race of a newborn. Sometimes, when queried, an observer's assessment of one's race is different from the self-definition of race. Moreover, individuals can consider themselves to be of multiple origins. Therefore, when designing your questions regarding race for a research study, allow respondents to choose all the categories of which they consider themselves a member.

Think

Because both race and ethnicity relate to social constructs that have varied throughout time and because there is increased mixing of populations throughout the world, some have suggested that social groupings of people should combine race and ethnicity into one common entity. What do you think? Others suggest that for purposes of identifying medically important characteristics, researchers could drop both race and ethnicity, and replace them with a few questions regarding ancestry. What do you think?

Ethnicity has also been described by researchers as being a social construct, but it is generally considered separate from race by sociologists. Ethnicity is a social construct based on identification with a particular culture and a shared group history. In the United States today, the most frequently used ethnic category is Hispanic, which refers to peoples whose cultural practices derived from Spain or Portugal. In countries throughout the world, there are considerable numbers of ethnic groups based on cultural practices. Moreover, such groupings tend to change over time.

After recording age and basic demographic information, there are often other patient-level characteristics that are important to report in comparative effectiveness research. Such variables may be valuable so that the readers of the research know whether the subjects within the study are similar to themselves (for patients) or to their patients (for clinicians). One group of such variables relates to health-relevant lifestyle factors such as dietary intake, body mass index, waist circumference, usual exercise, use of tobacco products, and alcohol intake. Another group of significant variables relates to the medical history of diseases and disorders, including when they first were diagnosed, treatment, and complications. Other important factors to include in many research studies relate to preventive medicine such as immunizations, use of various recommended screening practices, monitoring of blood pressure, assessment of cholesterol levels, and other factors related to the prevention and/or early detection of disease.

For many of these variables, there is no need to reinvent the wheel. You will find that researchers have already paved your way, and have considered how such questions should be asked. Moreover, the validity (whether the variable or instrument actually measures what it is supposed to measure) and reliability (reproducibility) of many variables have already been determined.

Listed below are several commonly used variables in medical research:

Alcohol Intake: Suppose you wish to include baseline information regarding each subject's use of alcoholic beverages. There are established validated instruments to do this and therefore, it is wise to examine these first. Use the scientific literature to find methods for collecting this information in which the questions have demonstrated both validity and reliability. For example, Pilkonis and colleagues created item banks for alcohol use for the Patient-Reported Outcomes Measurement Information System (Pilkonis, 2013). A common instrument used to detect abuse of alcohol beverages is called the CAGE questionnaire. It consists of four questions:

- Have you ever felt that you ought to cut down on your drinking?
- Have people annoyed you by criticizing your drinking?
- Have you ever felt bad or guilty about your drinking?
- Have you ever had a drink first thing in the morning to steady your nerves or to get rid of a hangover?

When administered to inpatients, the CAGE questionnaire has been shown to be a valid tool for assessing whether or not a person has a history of alcohol abuse.

Tobacco use: Smoking cigarettes represents another commonly assessed lifestyle factor in which the validity and reliability of measurements have been assessed. Often investigators wish to differentiate a person who has never smoked cigarettes from a person who has. While one could directly inquire regarding "ever" versus "never" use, a common way to differentiate this in clinical research is by the following question:

Discover
Go online and search for valid questionnaires for measuring alcohol use or some variant of this phrase. See if you have any trouble finding at least 10 different questionnaires (or instruments). Then try restricting the search to a particular subgroup such as adolescence or pregnancy.

- Have you smoked at least 100 cigarettes in your entire life?

It is not unusual for adolescents to try cigarettes at some point, so setting a minimal level ensures that the investigator does not combine people who tried a few cigarettes when young (and never smoked again) with people who continued smoking over time. It is also common to assess the duration of smoking. To do this, common questions used in research are:

- How old were you when you first started to smoke fairly regularly?
- Do you now smoke cigarettes every day, some days, or not at all?
- How long has it been since you quit smoking cigarettes?

The researcher may also want to assess the quantity of cigarettes smoked. Questions regarding quantity may be added to duration to provide greater detail regarding patterns of use:

- On the average, how many cigarettes do you now smoke a day?
- On how many of the past 30 days did you smoke a cigarette?
- On the average, when you smoked during the past 30 days, about how many cigarettes did you smoke a day?
- During the past 12 months, have you stopped smoking for more than one day because you were trying to quit smoking?

Check It Out
Go to the Centers for Disease Control and Prevention site regarding Smoking & Tobacco Use Surveys (http://www.cdc.gov/tobacco/data_statistics/surveys/index.htm). For each of the surveys, you can read each question that was asked on smoking. Try selecting the National Youth Tobacco Survey. Scroll down to where it says "2011 NYTS Questionnaire." You can download it and read through the questions. Feel free to look at some of the tobacco-related questions on the other surveys. Besides smoking cigarettes, sometimes the questions deal with other tobacco products such as chewing tobacco, or with tobacco-related exposures such as second-hand smoke.

Such questions are often used to estimate the intensity of cigarette use and, sometimes, are represented as pack-years of cigarettes, which measures both quantity and duration. A pack-year is equivalent to 20 cigarettes smoked each day for an entire year.

The World Health Organization has an online guide for structuring tobacco questions for surveys to be used either at the population (country) level or at the individual level (http://www.who.int/tobacco/surveillance/en_tfi_tqs.pdf).

Physical activity: There are also valid and reliable instruments to measure exercise and physical activity. In public health research and preventive medicine, such instruments are often used as potential predictors of a condition or disease. In comparative effectiveness research, physical activity and mobility can also be very useful outcomes. Moreover, there are instances in which investigators wish to report baseline characteristics of participants by physical activity and these measures may serve as useful descriptors of an individual's level of health.

There are several common approaches to measuring physical activity and these include self-reporting on questionnaires, observation of activities, and direct measurement of motion. For example, a cardiac stress test may be used to evaluate functioning during physical exertion. Physical therapists extensively employ various tests related to ambulation and balance, such as the six-minute walk test to assess performance in patients with heart failure or who have chronic respiratory disease. Self-reports through questionnaires are also used and some of the common questions can be seen at the Centers for Disease Control and Prevention site within the Behavioral Risk Factor Surveillance System (http://www.cdc.gov/brfss/questionnaires.htm). Examples of these physical activity questions include "Have you participated in 150 minutes or more of aerobic physical activity per week?" and "Have you participated in muscle strengthening exercises more than twice per week?"

Other researchers have been interested in a useful pragmatic screening question on physical activity that could be utilized in primary care. They found that a single question can validly capture physical activity of benefit to health (Milton 2013). This question is, "In the past week, on how many days have you done a total of 30 minutes or more of physical activity, which was enough to raise your breathing rate?"

Medical conditions: At the start of a research study, data regarding current medical conditions and the history of various conditions are also frequently reported. Such histories are available in electronic medical records and can be very valuable as baseline patient descriptors in research studies. The percentage of patients with diabetes or hypertension or other common diseases may be reported in the text or listed in a table. Often the research question itself in a particular study determines the medical conditions listed for the participants. Occasionally this information includes the duration of the disorder or the patient's age when first diagnosed. Fortunately, there are several national surveys online that provide examples of questions regarding standardized approaches to elicit information regarding medical conditions. For example, here are typical questions regarding high blood pressure:

1. Have you ever been told by a doctor, nurse, or other health professional that you have high blood pressure?
2. Are you currently taking medicine for your high blood pressure?

For some diseases, it is important to provide baseline information regarding family history of disease. Examples of family history questionnaires may be found in medical

Check It Out
Examples of questions regarding medical conditions are available online at the National Health Interview Survey (http://www.cdc.gov/nchs/nhis/quest_data_related_1997_forward.htm). Choose one of the survey questionnaires at this site and look through the questions within the section that ascertains Conditions. For example, one of the questions is, "Have you ever been told by a doctor or other health professional that you have a seizure disorder or epilepsy?" Feel free to browse through the questions. Note that there separate questionnaires for adults and children.

genetics (http://www.genome.gov/11510372). Note the depth of information regarding each relative.

Patient Registries

A patient registry is a system that contains health-related information on patients with a common condition or characteristic. Such databases may be very simple, while others are more sophisticated with electronic capture and follow-up over time. Registries may be formed by a medical specialty group because of the interest in a certain disease such as a registry of children with meningomyelocele or a registry of people with Lewy body dementia. Heritable diseases are often candidates for registries such as those initiated for people with hemophilia.

Registries can be formed on the basis of health rather than a particular disease; these too can be used for medical research. There have been initiatives to form health registries such as various women's health registries throughout the United States, as well as the UNC Health Registry to better study how to prevent disease (http://unchealthregistry.org/). There are registries of families with multiple births, including the Swedish Twin Registry (http://ki.se/ki/jsp/polopoly.jsp?d=9610&l=en) with approximately 85,000 twin pairs and is the largest such registry worldwide. Other twin registries include the Mid-Atlantic Twin Registry with more than 50,000 twin pairs (http://www.matr.vcu.edu/) and the Danish Twin Registry (http://www.sdu.dk/en/om_sdu/institutter_centre/ist_sundhedstjenesteforsk/centre/dtr) that contains data from nearly all the twin births in Denmark since 1870. Wow!

The basis of a registry may also be centered on procedures or exposures rather than disease. For example, there are registries of patients undergoing surgical procedures, such as the Society of Thoracic Surgeons National Database, the European Cardiac Surgical Registry, the Australian Society of Cardiac Surgeons, and the Canadian Joint Replacement Registry. There are registries of patients who have specific medical devices. The US Food and Drug Administration is in the process of building a National Medical Device Registry and a Unique Device Identification System for monitoring utilization and complications related to medical devices. There are registries in environmental health of people exposed to asbestos (National Asbestos Exposure Register at http://www.asbestossafety.gov.au). as well as registries of people exposed to high levels of radiation or toxins (http://www.publichealth.va.gov/docs/exposures/registry-evaluation-brochure.pdf). There are also

Explore
Go to the Cystic Fibrosis Foundation's site for their Patient Registry (http://www.cff.org/livingwithcf/qualityimprovement/patientregistryreport/). This registry has been in operation for more than 40 years. Download their latest Report and take a look at the types of information that they track. Can you envision how data from this registry could be used in comparative effectiveness research?

registries of people who share a common experience, such as survivors of a terrorist attack or survivors of a great natural disaster.

As a researcher, you should ask yourself a few initial questions regarding a registry. Is it a population-based registry? That is, is it a registry that includes nearly all individuals with a particular condition or exposure within a circumscribed region during a specific time period? Is it a registry formed from a wide network of providers or is it a registry at a single site with a few participants? These questions relate to external validity, or how well the people in the registry reflect all such persons in the population as a whole. Other important aspects to investigate are the length of time the registry participants were observed, the fluidity of the cohort (are many members frequently dropping out and others coming in), and details regarding the types of information collected.

Think
Suppose that you wanted to form a registry. What type of registry would it be? What potential benefits would there be in forming this registry? Now conduct an online search. Did you find that there are such registries or similar registries?

A registry has the potential for being very useful in comparative effectiveness research when the records are electronic and the registry contains some depth regarding the health information available. If there were an electronic registry of 32,000 individuals and data were available regarding their treatments and health-related services received over a five-year period, this database can provide a research structure and potentially generate meaningful information to members of the registry, as well as to patients and health professionals in general. Often a registry tends to be more useful if the data are collected consistently over a period of time. The data should have a measurable degree of accuracy; that is, there is reasonable incorporation of quality control with regard to data entry and management. There may be opportunities to input data directly from registry participants online. Often, such registries can be housed within an agency, foundation or network of providers, and these entities would provide the necessary support for maintaining and updating the registry.

Take A Look
At the Agency for Healthcare Research and Quality site, there is a Registry of Patient Registries (https://patientregistry.ahrq.gov/faq/). Wow—a registry of registries! See if you can find it. Look through the variety of registries listed (you might try the Structured Search tab near the top to see the categories).

Comparative effectiveness research is described as using real-world data. The real world is diverse and changing. Studies which explore the variation in health practices and policies across populations can be very informative. Large population-based longitudinal studies can provide strength of evidence in numbers, and may also provide opportunities for investigations within subgroups of people who may be either at greater risk—or lower risk—of particular outcomes. Sometimes the availability of wide networks provides a mechanism to address important questions that cannot be answered elsewhere. If used wisely, there are opportunities to better understand the health of a population as a whole and to define the detailed underlying elements necessary for driving individual health.

One of the purposes of comparative effectiveness research is to provide meaningful answers to patients' typical questions such as "Given my personal characteristics, conditions, and preferences, what should I expect will happen to me?" None of us can change our age, our genetic profile (well, not quite yet), or what happened to us in the past. So given who we are today, the hope is that the results of research will provide these answers.

7

The Place

Place has been an influential driver in spearheading comparative effectiveness research. Place has been critical in recognizing different patterns of services and variations in patient outcomes. Location has always been an important aspect of epidemiology, but its full relevance to clinical practice has come a century and a half after John Snow's recognition of the importance of place in the cholera epidemics in London. While the turning point in public health was recognized through the importance of where people lived in London in relationship to cholera deaths, it was the investigators behind the *Dartmouth Atlas of Health Care* in the United States that brought the relevance of place to the modern New World. Where you live greatly affects your health.

Spatial relationships were often thought to result from the dynamics of human variation on differential disease risk. While it could be that geospatial variation is due to the characteristics of the people who reside in those areas, it could also be the types of exposures and services that they receive which drive outcomes. Are treatments and practice patterns similar in all locations? The experience in the United States clearly demonstrates that this is not the case. Medical services often show variability in frequency, cost, and content. For example, in a study of 144 hospitals throughout the United States, there was variation between hospitals in the receipt of red blood cell transfusions in patients who underwent coronary artery bypass graft surgery (Maddux 2009). At some hospitals, no patients were given intraoperative red blood cell transfusions, while at other hospitals, 85.7% of the patients received such transfusions. It begs the question: Why? Why do some patients at certain hospitals not receive this therapy but, at other locations, most patients who underwent the same surgical procedure do? Is this therapy appropriate or not? When there are differences in treatment for the same procedure in patients with the same condition, comparative effectiveness research can be very informative in answering these questions.

Geographic differences in medical services have spawned hypotheses and created the impetus for further investigation. The availability of clinical data from geographically diverse areas can serve as a foundational resource for studies in hospital settings, ambulatory centers, and primary care networks.

> **Discover**
>
> Let's explore the Interactive Atlas of Heart Disease and Stroke (http://apps.nccd.cdc.gov/DHDSPAtlas/viewer.aspx). Once the application has loaded, select US map with county data. Go ahead and select some of the Health Indicators, Determinants of Health, or Health Services. What variation do you see? Did you find anything that you did not previously know? The Henry J. Kaiser Family Foundation (http://kff.org/) has a set of health-related maps in many areas that are relevant to comparative effectiveness research. Click on one of their major topics and notice that you can display data in tables and maps. Another site for the examination of comparative health is the County Health Rankings site (http://www.countyhealthrankings.org/). It contains health-related data by counties in the United States. Ranking for different health outcomes are illustrated by location and year. Try looking at some of the measures for your favorite states. The Robert Wood Johnson DataHub displays useful health information by geographic location (http://www.rwjf.org/en/research-publications/research-features/rwjf-datahub.html). It also has a nice player at the bottom of the map for displaying the differing geography over time.

Increasingly, more data are becoming available as health care systems and networks are created and electronic records become operationalized. Findings from such databases can illustrate the degree to which geographic patterns of patient-relevant outcomes correlate with practices and services.

Place as a Basis for the Comparators

Place is an especially important factor at this point in time in American history. With new health care policies underway, the structural elements of these changes yield opportunities for investigation. An example is the health insurance called Medicaid, which historically has provided coverage for low-income individuals in the United States and is administered at the state level. Coverage and eligibility has varied somewhat from state to state. With changes in health policy, so too are there changes in eligibility and coverage of services. Some states have chosen to expand Medicaid while others have not. For investigators in comparative effectiveness research, this provides an opportunity to look at differences in patient outcomes across states. Utilization of various services and their effects on the health of populations can be compared. An example of a comparative effectiveness research investigation of differences in Medicaid coverage was reported in the *New England Journal of Medicine* by Baicker and colleagues (Baicker, 2013). Because of a random lottery drawing of Oregon residents for inclusion into Medicaid, which occurred in 2008, the investigators were able to design a randomized controlled trial to compare people who did and did not receive Medicaid services (comparators) with various health outcomes within the first two years of enrollment. Health-related quality of life improved in those who received Medicaid, particularly in relationship to mental health with lower rates of depression. There were no significant improvements in physical health evident with Medicaid coverage in the first two years, although it did reduce financial hardship on the beneficiaries. Similar to this Oregon experiment, the state-level variation in Medicaid coverage with the new health policies provides an avenue for a natural experiment.

Geographic Information Systems

Information generated from using Geographic Information Systems (GIS) has signaled new opportunities to study health-relevant utilization of services and population outcomes. These systems provide a mechanism for inputting, storing, processing, and extracting geographic data. Often data are extracted from different sources and integrated for a wide range of applications.

Many of the GIS applications in health relate to public health. These can be especially useful for research regarding the distribution of infectious diseases or environmental exposures. There are applications with relevance to tracking infectious disease outbreaks, as well as for workforce issues related to lead abatement. GIS applications have been informative in studies related to geographic variation in rates of asthma and respiratory disease. Emergency services have been evaluated, as well as mechanisms for the prevention of injuries or violence. GIS may also be utilized for studies that investigate differences in access to health care or variation in outcomes due to health disparities. An example of geovisualization with ring maps was published showing racial disparity in diabetes prevalence (Stewart, 2011). Below are some examples of GIS health-related avenues for investigation:

- **Examining access to health services.** An example is a study that was conducted in Australia (Ranasinghe, 2012). The authors used an integrated data network containing information regarding the population, the hospitals, and the roads. They found that only 40% of the population had timely access to reperfusion services for ST-segment-elevation myocardial infarction. They then compared different approaches to mitigating this problem—for example, direct transport to primary percutaneous coronary intervention facilities improved access for 19% of the population, while optimizing medical service responses yielded only 2% improvement.
- **Examining variations in drug use.** There was an interesting systematic review in which the authors assembled all the GIS studies on prescription drug use (Wangia, 2013). They found that medication use was widely documented by geographical units (regions, states, postal codes, etc.), and much of it was captured by period prevalence (use on an annual basis, although monthly and daily were also available in some studies). There was also information on defined daily dose. The authors commented that, given the extensive research in small area variation generally, there were relatively few studies yet on drug use. This field holds potential for further investigations.
- **Health and the built environment.** There is increasing evidence that the built environment (including hospitals, clinics, and planned outdoor space) influences health outcomes. There are opportunities

in comparative effectiveness research to evaluate the effects of specific components of the built environment on patient-centered outcomes. Such studies have particular relevance when planning new health facilities or community areas that could potentially impact the quality of life. In addition, they can relate to the open structural environment that has particular importance in everyday life, such as spaces that make allowances for and encourage physical activity.

- **Emergency preparedness.** There are considerable opportunities to investigate the delivery of health services during natural disasters and emergency situations. Differing approaches on a regional or national level can be explored such as preventive approaches to personal safety and disaster mitigation. There may be opportunities for limited trials regarding the examination of different recovery approaches in situations where the benefit is not yet known. An example is a decision support system for the response to infectious-disease emergencies based on WebGIS and mobile services tested in China with potential applications in developing countries (Li, 2013).

- **Impact of the health care workforce.** Geographic information is available regarding characteristics of the workforce in health care, and variables include staffing levels and availability of certain providers. These distributions can be utilized to evaluate associations with patient outcomes and to plan head-to-head comparisons of policies or initiatives relevant to the workforce. These may have particular import for the coordination of care across different types of providers. An example of using geospatial information to explore the association between the availability of dentists and the rates of tooth decay and gum disease was published by Saman and colleagues (Saman, 2011)

- **Interventions to mitigate infectious disease outbreaks.** Infectious disease modeling is quite developed compared to other applications. Such modeling through space and time can be expanded to evaluate different approaches taken at regional, national, or international levels and the influence on seasonal patterns and epidemic situations. If you are interested in public health applications, the Centers for Disease Control and Prevention provide a GIS section (http://www.cdc.gov/gis/).

- **Identifying and targeting areas for screening.** There have been several applications of using geospatial data to identify areas where people at greater risk of disease are not yet receiving preventive screening measures at desired levels. Sometimes linking

---

Explore

Go to the Dartmouth Atlas of Health Care online (http://www.dartmouthatlas.org/). Examine some of the data available by region or by topic. Select a few options and see how utilization of services and health outcomes vary throughout the country. There are several basic geographic areas that are often used to visualize data in the Atlas:

- HRR: Hospital Referral Regions
- HSA: Hospital Service Areas
- PCSA: Primary Care Service Areas

See if you can find some analyses that utilize each of these areas.

the characteristics that define high risk with screening adherence on a geographic level is informative and can lead to specific interventions (Lofters, 2013). Such applications can link appropriate providers with patients.

These are a few possible applications. You may well be aware of others or may discover additional applications as they emerge. An excellent example of the marriage between health and geography is the *Dartmouth Atlas of Health Care*. Health services data are available across geographic areas in the United States. For example, Medicare data were utilized to assess the frequency of various types of surgical procedures for patients who reside in circumscribed hospital service areas and hospital referral regions.

There also can be geographic boundaries that occur because of the structure of health care systems in local and regional areas. Networks of health care providers can serve as boundaries. For many years, the Mayo Clinic has provided services to the residents in the community of Rochester, Minnesota, and the health care statistics generated from this area have been very informative. The structure of provider networks can form the basis of geographic studies, and the distribution of particular types of providers (such as hospice providers) can form the basis of geographic analyses.

Place at the Individual Level

Take A Look
Examine the variety of geographic information systems available throughout the world that may have relevance to health. Explore the Global Health Observatory Map Gallery (http://gamapserver.who.int/maplibrary/) and take a look at some of the available maps and information. HealthMap is another site that is worth investigating. It provides outbreak data and real-time surveillance. Another related site in the HealthMap Vaccine Finder (http://flushot.healthmap.org/). This site helps people find available vaccines and provides information regarding vaccine recommendations. While you might not initially see the connection between a vaccine finder and comparative effectiveness research, keep an open mind. Such informational sites could well serve as comparators in such studies.

Explore
The geographic distribution of people with specific cancers has been studied, and summary information is available at the National Cancer Institute including an overview of geographic information systems and science (http://gis.cancer.gov/). Datasets are available, as well as tools, plug-ins, and open-access software. Mapping capabilities and mechanisms for the generation of graphs and tables are available. It may be worthwhile to take the time to read the Overview anad explore the NCI GIS Portal. Cancer mortality maps are readily available (http://ratecalc.cancer.gov/), and the underlying data are downloadable. Examination of the variation in cancer incidence, mortality, and services may be useful for studies evaluating health policies.

Comparative effectiveness research can be enhanced through evaluation of therapies and services across regions, but location can also be important from the perspective of the individual patient. For example, comparators may involve obtaining the patient's opinion on where he or she would like events to occur. This is the essence of patient-centered outcomes. Approximately 70% of Americans would prefer to die in their own homes, but only 33% of them actually do (Teno, 2013). Why?

> **Explore**
>
> There are many studies that utilize defined small geographical units as the basis of investigation. Zip codes are either five or nine digit codes used by the US Postal Service for delivering mail. Zip codes loosely identify geographic areas, but are specific for a post office or delivery station (rather than residents' homes). The US Census Bureau took these zip codes and estimated their geographic location to greater precision; such codes are called ZIP Code Tabulation Areas (ZTCAs). Since these have an exact latitude and longitude, they can be mapped and linked with other geographic data. Search for US Census Data Mapper (http://www.census.gov/geo/maps-data/maps/datamapper.html). Launch the Mapper and explore the options. Take a look at the geographic patterns for various options.

Some patients—especially those with mobility problems or disabilities—would prefer to have a house call for a medical visit rather than having to arrange transportation to a clinic setting. Being able to receive certain types of services at specific locations can form the foundation of comparators used in comparative effectiveness research. The incorporation of one-stop shopping for medical services, especially in commonly visited drug stores or supermarkets, is another avenue for research. The availability of health personnel in particular locations, such as school nurses and their effect on the wellness of children, is a significant issue for further exploration. This is especially important as certain chronic illnesses become more common in children, such as asthma, autism, and obesity.

Elements of place from the perspective of the individual can be important in the design of comparative effectiveness research in several ways:

- **The importance of place in designing patient-centered research.** In comparative effectiveness research, the desires of the patient may influence the intent of the study. For example, the availability of hospice services may be valuable for terminally ill patients, and therefore studies can be designed to compare interventions which reach this objective. Geographic variation in hospices and its relation to community factors has been explored (Silveira, 2011).
- **The importance of place in structuring the comparators.** Sometimes place can be an integral part of the intervention. Whether blood pressure is measured at home or whether it is measured during office visits can define the structure of an intervention (Rogers, 2001). Remote monitoring of blood pressure, in which patients record their blood pressure at home and the readings are sent electronically to clinicians, can be compared with approaches using blood pressure taken during clinic visits.
- **The importance of place in the definition of the outcome.** The outcome may also be defined by place. Being able to return to work after surgery may be a relevant patient-centered outcome. Hospital readmission is a frequently used outcome measure in research; 30-day readmission rates are standard outcomes for assessing the quality of care. Being able to avoid another hospital visit is often an important outcome for patients.

8

The Time

While we live in the present, researchers spend considerable time studying the past in order to predict the future. Predicting the future is an interesting exercise. For example, there is a model by EarthRisk Technologies that can predict the weather 40 days before it occurs. The model is based on big data—60 years of weather pattern data chugging through 82 billion calculations. What if we could accurately predict health outcomes in patients 40 days in advance? Well, we can do this now—a bit crudely. But with additional data, our predictions have the potential to be more precise and provide greater clarity regarding specific long-term outcomes. Do you think that we will ever attain the ability to predict health and disease over a ten-year period? Or, perhaps, a lifespan?

Time is integral to health and is reflected in fundamental relationships. You may have already recognized some of these patterns. Overall mortality risk tends to follow a J-shaped pattern by age in populations. The times prior to and just after birth tend to be risky, not only in terms of mortality, but with other disorders as well. Birth is a time in which developmental irregularities or problems during delivery can play a role in adapting to the new environment. Once we progress into the middle childhood years, overall mortality tends to be rather low and, as years of adulthood progress, various chronic diseases generally increase impacting mortality. If one pinpoints particular diseases or injuries, age (i.e., time since birth) may pretty well define the problem. Many disorders are quite age-specific. Some disorders and injuries track higher during adolescence and young adulthood. In fact, seasoned researchers and clinicians can take any slice of the population and do a fairly good prediction regarding the age of this slice by just knowing the health behaviors and disorders present in that particular age group. Anorexia nervosa? Likely to be females aged 12 to 25 years.

There are different aspects of time that are important to consider when planning comparative effectiveness research. Time considerations are essential when developing conceptual models of the hypotheses, selecting the participants, planning the intervention, measuring the outcomes, and conducting the analyses.

Time Considerations with the Outcome

Time is a critical component of evaluating outcomes. In comparative effectiveness research, outcomes may reflect the level of functioning, improvement in capabilities, and various health-related states that influence one's ability to perform the necessary tasks of everyday life. All of these are time-sensitive.

Pain, for example, is a common outcome in clinical research. Within the Patient Reported Outcomes Measurement Information System (http://www.nihpromis.org/), there are measures related to pain interference, physical health, anxiety, depression, fatigue, sleep disturbance, social function, and global health. One of the pediatric questions is:

- In the past seven days, I had trouble sleeping when I had pain.
  - Never
  - Almost never
  - Somewhat
  - Often
  - Almost always

Specification of a relevant time period (e.g., in the past seven days) is crucial, since the outcome itself can change over time.

The element of time for constructing basic measures of health outcomes is incorporated as a core principle in epidemiology. So, for the seven-day time period listed above, we would call this "period prevalence"—a measurement of what occurred in a fixed period of time. The amount of time used for period prevalence depends upon the specific entity being measured. For some food frequency questionnaires, such periods can be stipulated as "over the last month" or "over the last three months." On the 36-Item Short Form Health Survey, there are items that require an assessment of what occurred in the past four weeks.

Period prevalence is often distinguished from point prevalence, which is an assessment of what occurred at a particular point in time or, for some real-time assessments, what is occurring right now. For example, one of the patient-reported outcomes measurements on physical health is:

- Are you able to walk a block on flat ground?
  - Without any difficulty
  - With a little difficulty
  - With some difficulty
  - With much difficulty
  - Unable to do

This measures current ability to perform a specific task. Outcomes that assess one's ability to do an activity at a particular point in time reflect point prevalence. Technically, there is a little bit of wiggle room between point prevalence and period prevalence because it takes time to perform an activity and time, itself, can be measured very precisely. But for most health applications, the difference is noticeable and, in any instance, it is important that the investigators state the specific point in time or the period of time utilized when describing their study (in the methods section).

In real life, it is not uncommon that there is some complexity in the use of time for certain health measures. This may occur as a consequence of the natural history of the disease. Take the process of infection as an example. This is a frequently used outcome in research, and with a little reflection, one realizes that it can be more difficult to measure than at first glance. There is an incubation period during which one is exposed to infectious organisms but you do not yet experience any symptoms. Then there is a period in which the first symptoms may appear (called a prodrome), which may be fleeting or last several days (the prodromal period). The period of communicability is the time period in which you could readily pass these pathogens to others; this sometimes occurs before and sometimes after symptoms are evident, depending upon the particular type of infectious agent. After symptoms occur, there may be a series of stages with a progression of different symptoms until resolution and recovery. In research, we often measure whether or not an infection occurred. This is an appropriate outcome because the process itself and its associated symptoms are important to people. However, it is still possible to refine such outcomes with more granularity so as to measure the effect of the infection on the functioning of patients throughout the infectious process, to examine elements of the process to further explore disease transmission, or measure the complications of the infection and the lingering functional effects of infection.

There is another critical aspect of time that is inherent in the measurement of outcomes. It becomes noticeable when examining particular examples such as breast cancer. Say we had a mechanism for assessing the prevalence of breast cancer. We surveyed a random sample of the entire population and asked this question, "Have you ever been told by a doctor or other health professional that you have breast cancer?" If we summarized the answers from all the survey participants, we would be obtaining the prevalence of that type of cancer at a given point in time (when the survey was performed). This prevalence is actually a reflection of many underlying occurrences. For example, this prevalence does not reflect all people who were ever diagnosed with this disease, because some may have already died. The incidence of disease or the rate in which new events occur in a population is a better reflection of all such occurrences—capturing both those persons who are living after receiving this diagnosis and those who have died. A different way to think of this outcome is in terms of one's risk over their entire lifetime. If we observed people over their entire lives, what is the likelihood that they would develop breast cancer? For American women, the chances are about one in eight. Or, one could use the probability of occurrence during the next 10 years, given that a patient is now at a certain age. Since comparative effectiveness research is broad in its approach, keep in mind the possibility of various time-sensitive measures and how you would like to best capture the essence of the outcome in the context of a study.

There are several options for dealing with time issues relevant to the outcome:

- If it is important to assess changes in the outcome or to ascertain extended abilities over time, the outcome can be measured repeatedly. So if the outcome is the 10 Meter Walk Test (i.e., the speed at which one walks 10 meters), one can measure this once a week for 12 weeks. You can also choose to measure this outcome before the intervention so that you have a baseline measurement (or series of baseline measurements), and then repeatedly record the outcome after the start of the intervention.
- If the outcome is acute, the investigator can measure the occurrence as a binary event (yes or no), and also the time in which it occurred. Capturing both the event and the time of the event allows more flexibility in the analyses. Survival analyses are often utilized to take into account time-to-event and offer important details regarding timing from the initiation of the comparators to the time when the outcome occurred.
- If progression of outcomes develops gradually, there may be various milestones of accomplishment that are important to chronicle over time. Occasionally the outcomes occur in a natural progression— being able to sit up at the side of the bed, being able to stand up independently, being able to walk within a room, and being able to walk outside for several hours may form a natural progression showing improvement over time.
- With the use of patient-centered outcomes, there is an opportunity to incorporate time from the perspective of the patient. The amount of time spent doing specific activities may be very important. The researcher can either record the amounts of time spent on various activities or directly ask individuals questions that reflect the value of their time. This may involve an examination of time-relevant measures that constitute preference during ones' daily life or of the quality of life for individuals with serious illness or advanced age.
- For some large national and international studies, time is incorporated into the outcome measure itself. Examples include healthy life years and disability-adjusted life years (DALY). These can be important indicators of health for an entire population.
- Longitudinal databases can serve an important role in ascertainment of outcomes over a long period of time. Randomized trials tend to be expensive, and often do not follow patients for 20 or 30 years

after enrollment. However, large linked databases can be utilized to assess different types of long-term outcomes and may be useful in the evaluation in the effects of therapies.

Time Considerations in Study Design

During the process of study design, time is an important consideration for the following elements.

During selection of participants. Subject selection in prospective comparative effectiveness research studies involves an evaluation of the number of possible subjects who can be enrolled within a certain time period. This frequently involves enrollment that continues throughout a defined time period in the study. If there is seasonal variation or other variants in the mechanisms involved with recruitment (e.g., frequency of clinic visits), these should be evaluated to develop the necessary tools to facilitate enrollment.

For retrospective longitudinal studies on large numbers of patients from electronic databases, there can be some flexibility in selection. When databases contain several years of data, the time period used to define subject selection is often dictated more by the frequency at which the outcome occurs. If the outcome is common, the investigator may need a year or two of data in order to answer the research question. If the outcome is rare, 20 years of data may be necessary. Such time considerations are important for calculating the number of study subjects necessary to detect the outcome measurements that are of interest.

During implementation of the interventions. Sometimes the intervention is not a one-time occurrence, but a change in behavior that is expected to continue. Thus the measurement of such interventions should encompass different elements related to the continuity of such behavioral changes over time. Adherence to therapies, such as adherence to a particular medication regimen, can be assessed at various time points, and the effects of specific patterns of behavior can be discerned. Variations in such behavior can constitute a very important aspect of study.

Study design may be built around time considerations integral to subject assignment to therapies. Examples would include the crossover trial and the stepped wedge trial designs in which patients are assigned to different comparators at different times. In a typical crossover trial, it is the timing (or the sequence) of the treatment that is randomized. The first patient may be assigned first to treatment A and then to treatment

> **Plan**
> There is considerable interest, from both physicians and patients, regarding the average time of a typical doctor's visit. Suppose that you were to use this interest to develop interventions relevant to this time for purposes of comparative effectiveness research. First, search online to obtain some general perspective on this issue from the general public. You might try searching for average time with doctor (or related terms). Then think about how you could possibly use this interest to build comparators in a study. Would you develop tools to help patients prepare for the visit? Would you develop alternative adjunct mechanisms by which patients and doctors could communicate? Would you evaluate whether there were some procedures or tools that could by used by physicians to enhance the visit? The field is wide open. What are your ideas?

B, while another patient may be assigned first to treatment B and then to treatment A. In a typical stepped wedge trial, groups of patients are assigned to various treatments at different times with the sequence or timing of the treatments incorporated into the trial design.

A different issue regarding time is whether to target the intervention at particular times when the individuals are most at risk. This occurs in many research studies. Investigators target certain therapies or services to those populations at the time period when they most (likely) need it. Interventions in toddlers to improve preschool development or in adolescents to reduce teenage pregnancy are targeted to certain time periods in life. There may also be increased efforts to target particular time periods in life that may be more challenging—the time period after the death of a spouse or child, the time period after major surgery, or the time period after diagnosis of Huntington's chorea. While some periods for targeted interventions may be straightforward to spot, there can also be greater consideration for time periods that may greatly impact the quality of life.

Time Measures in Clinical Research

There are certain measures in clinical research that have historically been incorporated because of opportunity and application to practice. Often researchers have records of procedures, diagnoses, and occurrences during hospitalizations. Thus, in-hospital mortality is a common outcome seen in the medical literature. In clinical research, there are a few time-related measures that are commonly used and are of particular note:

- **Hospital length of stay** tends to be a very skewed measure. There are many patients who stay in hospital for a few days or so. For example, in the United States in year 2010, the median length of stay for all hospitalizations was three days (http://hcupnet.ahrq.gov/). However, there are also some patients who stay in hospital for a very long time—sometimes years. Because of this, the probability of observing a certain outcome (for example, infection) may be very different in a patient who stays in hospital for three days compared to a patient who stays for 42 days. In terms of a research study in which investigators compare patients undergoing two different procedures, using in-hospital occurrence of events sometimes poses problems because of these different observation times. You could imagine that those patients who do well after surgery and are discharged within three days after surgery may be relatively healthy compared to those patients who stay in the hospital weeks after the surgery because of complications. These inconsistencies in follow-up after an intervention could have important consequences regarding the interpretation of the results. If there were an opportunity to observe patients for a consistent time period (e.g., from the date of the surgery to 30 days after surgery), everyone in the study would have a similar period in which to evaluate the outcome.

- **In-hospital mortality** is another commonly used outcome in clinical studies. It too has some underlying complexities that warrant mentioning. The hospitalization itself does not always capture the entire episode of care for a patient. That is, it might not constitute all the contiguous health care services related to therapy for a specific illness for a patient. Sometimes patients are discharged to a skilled nursing facility or a rehabilitation center for further treatment. Sometimes patients are followed by home health services after hospital discharge. At first glance, one might expect that occurrences in an acute care hospital might capture any fatalities due to procedures received during hospitalization, but it is not uncommon for some patients, depending upon their age and condition, to die after hospital discharge. Therefore the in-hospital mortality rate (the proportion of hospitalized patients who died) can be calculated and is often seen in the medical literature, but the underlying dynamics should always be kept in mind. For researchers who have the ability to link various health files, sometimes it is possible to calculate the actual cumulative mortality rate for a fixed length of time. With merging hospital files with other data (e.g., the National Death Index), one could determine the 30-day mortality rate after the date of a given procedure. This may provide a more consistent approach to observation for all the patients who underwent that particular procedure.

Time Considerations with Increased Use of Technology

In addition to providing health care that is effective and safe, another consideration is timeliness of services. There are expanding opportunities to incorporate technologies that provide information in a more timely fashion. For example, **point-of-care testing** of glucose, electrolytes, coagulation markers, drugs, infectious agents, and a host of other medically useful markers in blood, urine, saliva, and other tissues is available. Point-of-care testing can be important comparators in comparative effectiveness research. For example, point-of-care testing for home-bound patients can be compared with testing during clinic visits for the effects on outcomes. The investigator can evaluate whether providing information more rapidly and by this particular mechanism impacts the trajectories of functioning and utilization of other services. The researcher can also assess whether increased point-of-care testing with rapid incorporation into the electronic medical record impacts inpatient outcome as compared with reduced point-of-care testing (i.e., incorporation at a later time, generally after hospital discharge). Anticipated benefits of point-of-care testing as well as possible risks (such as increased likelihood of infection through repeated testing) could be examined. In addition, increased patient education regarding test results may be feasible in a point-of-care study and could serve as a possible comparator (i.e., linking point-of-care education with point-of-care testing). These circumstances can form the basis of important studies in comparative effectiveness research.

Explore

Comb the Web to find an example of an interesting technology that could potentially be relevant to point-of-care testing and health. Can you imagine a way in which this technology could be utilized in the context of a comparative effectiveness study?

9

The Fit

One of the finest talents of a researcher is to be able to design a good study that answers a specific question regarding an important issue. After the study elements are conceptualized and decisions regarding the hypothesis are finalized, the next step is to marry the hypothesis with a suitable design. Researchers who repeatedly go through this process develop insight.

First, you should know that it is possible to design different studies for the same hypothesis. In fact, this happens quite often. An investigator may choose one design, but another investigator would have designed it a bit differently. Does that mean that one researcher was correct and the other wrong? Not necessarily. With human research, a researcher's particular access to various populations or patient groups may be very influential in how the studies are designed. Not everyone has the same set of circumstances to begin with, and therefore, a variety of approaches is common. In fact, looking at a research question from different angles is a good thing.

Consider possible choices for study design for original research studies. While reviews are important, keep in mind that systematic reviews are totally dependent upon the quality of the underlying original research studies under examination. It is the well-conducted original research study that is of utmost importance. These are the generators of new knowledge and form the foundation of new scientific evidence. The ability for researchers to design new studies to answer important questions is central to helping people make informed health decisions.

While it may be relatively straightforward for experienced researchers to narrow the choices of study designs for a particular hypothesis, it helps to go through examples when you are first starting. Let's examine a few situations.

Designs in Primary Care Settings

The primary care setting can form the backbone of efforts to make peoples' lives better. This is the usual setting for an intersection between a person with a health problem and a health care provider. This setting may offer many opportunities for explorations into what works and what doesn't for most people. It is here where many problems are first addressed—a headache, a twisted ankle, a nasty cough, this itchy rash, feeling anxious, can't sleep at night, a stomach ache—in other words, all the everyday issues that people sometimes deal with on their own but for which they often need help. Moreover, such issues may forecast something more serious.

There are a variety of designs that may be used in primary care settings. Some designs are more rigorous and provide more definitive evidence of an effect. For example, randomized trials using large numbers of subjects tend to provide better evidence for or against an effect. Let's start with an important rule of thumb:

> **RULE OF THUMB:** When selecting a design, consider the most rigorous designs first.

If ethical and feasible, consider randomization in the primary care setting. Do not toss this important design feature out the window too quickly. You would be surprised at the willingness of individuals to undergo randomization for certain interventions. Of course, your decision should always be based on the mandatory requirements guiding the conduct of human subjects research. But when your hypothesis is formed and you are considering randomization with specific comparators, look to the existing medical literature for randomized trials with similar comparators. Were there other investigators who were able to randomize people to such treatments? Discuss with colleagues the challenges posed by doing this. However, there are times when randomization cannot be performed. There may be comparators that are of interest for a specific outcome, but the comparator may be unethical to use because of its known health risks in other areas. A careful and thorough assessment of when and which types of patients may benefit is necessary before deciding the study design.

In the primary care setting, individual information is available and this provides an opportunity for capturing background information and observing individuals over time. Below are some options:

- **Randomized trial with comparators**. When randomization is possible, there are several trial designs that may be suitable. The cluster randomized trial is a natural choice when the therapies can be administered over a large number of clinics or practices. When providers from a network of practices demonstrate interest in a research project, random assignment of clinics or practices may be a good fit for examining patient effects in the primary care setting. The randomized stepped wedge trial is often a good choice when it is more feasible to implement the interventions in stages over time. Depending upon the research questions, you may also consider some of the pragmatic adaptive randomized trial designs that allow flexibility.

For studies with multiple comparators in which there is an interest in interactive effects, you may consider a randomized factorial design.

- **Within-person trial**. A randomized N-of-1 trial in primary care is a natural extension of clinical practice. This approach can provide information regarding the question, "What's best for me?" The knowledge that is gained from participating in an N-of-1 trial is directly applicable to decision making regarding the patient's choices of therapies, and therefore has a possibility of improving his or her own health. Furthermore, for therapies in which there is a natural comparator site within an individual (right/left appendage, right/left eye, right/left ear, etc.), a split body trial could be used, which also allows a within-person comparison.
- **Nonrandomized trial**. For those therapies or interventions that cannot be randomized due to ethical or feasibility issues, the investigators could still conduct a trial without the randomization. In a clinic setting, this may be a practical approach. Clinicians may be administering the therapy anyway—and they could do so in the context of a trial. Often baseline information on all patients is available. The advantage of a trial, as opposed to an observational design, is the ability to offer preplanned consistent comparators in each study arm. The investigators can also arrange for consistent time-specific measurements of the outcome.
- **Longitudinal study**. When a trial is not feasible, there are a variety of observational longitudinal designs that are available. This is a very attractive choice when large electronic databases of patient-level data are available across many sites. If information regarding therapies, diagnoses, procedures, and meaningful outcomes is accessible, there are methods to structure these data elements into a formal design. As for any other study, a conceptual model should first be constructed relevant to the hypotheses of interest. Often, the best approach is to recreate what occurred longitudinally in patients so that the temporal sequence of events can be identified.

Think
In the United States, the Institute of Medicine developed a list of Initial National Priorities for Comparative Effectiveness Research (http://www.iom.edu/Reports/2009/ComparativeEffectivenessResearchPriorities.aspx). The pdf is free. Look over some of the priorities that may be related to primary care. For example, one of the priorities is to compare the effectiveness of mindfulness-based interventions (e.g., yoga, meditation, deep breathing training) and usual care in treating anxiety and depression, pain, cardiovascular risk factors, and chronic diseases. Think about how you could possibly design a study to address this issue. Select any of the other primary care-related priorities and think about possible design options.

There are other choices that have been used in primary care settings so keep an open mind when weighing the different options. Sometimes a good review of the literature will spark an idea for a different approach.

Designs in Institutionalized Settings

Hospitals and skilled nursing facilities are important settings in which to evaluate the effectiveness of various procedures and therapies. Often patients are critically ill or have serious chronic conditions, and therefore the feasibility of randomization must be judiciously considered. In particular, issues with cognition and the ability of patients to consent to participation are important factors. Yet it is also important to have rigorous evidence so that therapies can be improved for hospitalized patients. In order to do so, comparative studies of possible therapeutic options may be informative. Below are some designs that are useful in institutionalized settings:

- **Randomized trial with comparators**. There are several trial designs that would be useful to consider. Multisite randomized trials with active comparators are the mainstay for definitive evidence in this regard and, when necessary, the use of pragmatic adaptive features could be examined. Cluster randomized trials and stepped wedge designs are an option when there is a large network of facilities for implementation. These can work well for instances in which new health initiatives are planned for implementation at the group level (e.g., intensive care units, hospitals within a consortium). A stepped wedge design can be a practical approach, because it may be easier to implement new practices over a gradual time period than to start them all simultaneously.
- **Nonrandomized trial**. If randomization is not an option, nonrandomized comparisons of therapies for those comparators that would naturally involve patient choice are a possibility. Keep important design elements such as blind assessment of the outcome when feasible, and incorporate consistent assessments of baseline characteristics, choice of and compliance with selected comparators, and patient-reported outcomes. A trial may yield a clearer distinction between the choices than sole observation because the choices can be more structured and monitored, with consistent administration. It can also provide an opportunity to incorporate specifically planned patient-reported outcomes similar to randomized trials.
- **Cohort study**. In institutional settings, there is considerable detail regarding the patient's status, medications, procedures, laboratory tests, and other relevant clinical data during the entire stay. Therefore, a longitudinal study of hospitalized patients using electronic clinical databases is a natural choice. If all of the data are not available electronically, additional information can be retrieved from the patient's hardcopy chart. Such studies are strengthened by utilizing data across many different hospitals; consortium data are sometimes available. There are instances in which hospital data may

be linked with other complementary databases and such longitudinal information may form the foundation for several comparative effectiveness studies.

- **Interrupted time series design.** When there are hospital policies or procedures that have changed over time, such "interrupters" can serve as an opportunity to assess effect. Evaluations of patient outcomes over time are routinely monitored for quality control purposes in a hospital setting and pre- to post-policy assessments are not uncommon. There may be instances in which you would prefer to evaluate these pre-post differences in the context of a research study (with human subjects' approval) and to include several comparators. Such evaluations can utilize group measures of effect (by unit or floor) if desired.
- **Case-crossover study.** In some instances it is possible to conduct case-crossover studies in a hospital setting for more rare outcomes. Hospitalizations in which an event of interest occurred would constitute the cases (i.e., index hospitalizations). Hospitalizations from the same patients in which this event did not occur would constitute the comparison group (comparator hospitalizations). These are retrospective studies using electronic data of hospitalizations recorded over a certain time period, generally several years. For example, your outcome may be a hospitalization in which deep vein thrombosis developed during the stay. This would be your index hospitalization. Then, for the same patient, the hospitalizations in which deep vein thrombosis did not develop are the comparators. The research question is, "Why did the patient develop a venous blood clot during this hospitalization when he or she did not develop it in the other hospitalizations?" It is a within-person comparison, so there is strong control over many potential confounders.

Think
Revisit the Institute of Medicine's list of Initial National Priorities for Comparative Effectiveness Research (http://www.iom.edu/Reports/2009/ComparativeEffectivenessResearchPriorities.aspx). Find a few priorities that may be related to care in hospitalized patients or residents of skilled nursing facilities. For example, one of the priorities is to compare the effectiveness of robotic assistance surgery and conventional surgery for common operations, such as prostatectomies. What are some design options for this priority? Can you find other priorities related to hospitalization? If you, a friend, or a family member has ever experienced a hospitalization, do you have any other suggestions for a research priority based on your experiences?

Designs for Emergency Services

Emergency services are often thought of as happening in an emergency department within a hospital. While this certainly occurs, there are other settings in which emergency services are received by individuals. These include ambulances and helicopters in emergency transit; sites involved in search and rescue operations during natural disasters or accidents; and homes, workplaces, and community locales in which assistance has been requested or is required from fire department personnel, police, and emergency medical crews. It also includes an array of services that are associated with crisis situations such as those provided by poison control professionals, lifeguards, suicide prevention specialists, and international teams providing disaster or famine relief.

The application of research to such diverse settings may, at times, be challenging but has been achieved by many investigators. While there are situations when life and death hang in the balance and in which actions may require quick decisions, there are also settings where health professionals can work to evaluate differences in patient outcomes and to improve practices whenever possible. Below are some possible options for study design:

- **Randomized trial with comparators**. At first glance, one might think that randomization would never be possible in an emergency situation, but there are instances where randomization is feasible and ethical. Consideration of pragmatic adaptive trials would be an option, particularly because emergency situations can involve unpredictability and incorporating some flexibility may be prudent. You may wish to consider a sequential trial that is terminated as soon as a significant effect is observed.

- **Nonrandomized trial**. If randomization is not an option, nonrandomized comparisons of therapies could be considered. The investigators could capture information regarding patient-reported outcomes whenever possible. That is, patients could be observed over time to access their health and functioning after the immediate emergency situation has passed. Comparators could be clearly defined and consistently measured.

- **Longitudinal designs**. When registries or large electronic databases are available, longitudinal studies may be informative regarding the types of outcomes experienced across a wide range of patients, as well as for more rare outcomes. When there are large databases in which populations are observed over time and data regarding emergency services (and the dates of such services) are available, this may serve as a valuable opportunity to study the factors that preceded the emergency or to investigate the long-term outcomes after emergency procedures were performed. Linking of databases could allow examination across regions or countries.

Search

Go to PubMed Clinical Queries (http://www.ncbi.nlm.nih.gov/pubmed/clinical) and and search for "(randomized AND trial AND "emergency department"[Title/Abstract])". On the left-hand side, you will see the Clinical Study Categories. Select the category Prognosis and the scope Narrow. Look at the different types of randomized trials related to emergency services that relate to the prognosis of patients. See anything of interest? Go ahead and explore related searches such as Therapy, Diagnosis or Etiology.

Designs for Home Health Services

Home health services are often beneficial after hospital discharge or when intermittent skilled nursing care, physical therapy, or speech therapy is necessary for recovery. Studies may include interventions to encourage self-management in certain domains such as nutrition or mobility, as well as interventions that address the process of care such as telehealth applications and methods to coordinate care. Outcomes can be patient reported. Because the patients are in a home setting, the researcher has an opportunity to collect observations of daily living directly from patients or through examination by the visiting health professional. For example, studies involving postpartum home visits after labor and delivery have been conducted in order to assess both maternal and infant outcomes.

There are fewer investigations of home health services in the medical literature than research conducted in clinical settings. Few have been trials. Part of the lack of studies may be due to the diverse structures of home health agencies and the feasibility of implementation. There are home health agency electronic databases available from the Centers for Medicare and Medicaid Services that include patient-level variables in older adults, which could be of potential interest in comparative effectiveness research studies.

Search

Go to PubMed and search for "visiting nurses" OR "home visits" (http://www.ncbi.nlm.nih.gov/pubmed). Examine the types of studies that have been published. You might try a few other search filters that may narrow your search to a topic of interest to you. Do you see any original research studies? If so, what was their design?

Designs for Screening

There are two broad categories of research related to disease detection. The first poses the question, "Does this test accurately identify people who truly have the condition and accurately identify the people who truly do not have the condition?" Such diagnostic studies are common in the medical literature, and they usually involve the choice of a gold standard for determining what truly defines the diagnosis and what does not. This research employs particular statistics that define concepts such as positive predictive value of the test (how well a positive test predicts the disease) and can provide meaningful information regarding new tests versus a robust gold standard, when such a standard is available.

However, comparing a new test to a gold standard does not reach the goal of determining whether a specific test improves patient outcomes. Assessment of effectiveness is at the core of comparative effectiveness research. Therefore, a second category of research related to disease detection would be to compare specific screening tests with what eventually happened to the patient later on. Since screening tests are given to individuals who are asymptomatic and have early-stage (yet unrecognized) disease, the intent of using screening tests is to discover whether the early detection of disease leads to a longer, healthier life. Comparative effectiveness research provides a mechanism to assess patient outcomes when different screening approaches are used.

In summary, for studies of diagnosis or screening purposes there are two common major categories often seen in the medical literature:

- **Studies to assess the accuracy of a diagnostic or screening test.** These studies generally compare a diagnostic or screening test with a gold standard (definitive measurements or procedures indicating the absence or presence of that particular disease). Diagnostic tests are given to patients who have symptoms, while screening tests are given to patients with early disease without symptoms. Results are often reported as sensitivity, specificity, and predictive value, which reflect the discriminatory abilities of the test. They can be very valuable in assessing the accuracy of various tests. These studies evaluate the degree to which a test detects a condition; they do not measure whether the test actually benefits the patient in the long run.
- **Studies to assess the effectiveness of screening.** These studies are meant to evaluate whether a screening test benefits (or harms) people over the long term. These are generally randomized controlled trials or longitudinal studies that compare various screening approaches for particular diseases. Often the endpoint will be mortality, disease-free survival, or years of healthy life. Occasionally decision analysis or simulation approaches can be used to compare screening approaches as well.

Consider
It is important that you recognize the difference between these two types of studies often seen in the medical literature. The purpose, comparators, and outcomes are different. Go to one of the medical literature databases such as PubMed and search for "screening sensitivity specificity." Look at the structure of a few studies that evaluate accuracy of testing. Now search for "effectiveness of screening," and look at a few studies that evaluate the effectiveness of specific tests or approaches. Do you see some differences?

The Guide to Clinical Preventive Services is a manual that summarizes the medical evidence regarding screening tests and other preventive services. In the methods sections, there are separate categories that (a) report the medical evidence regarding the accuracy of the test and (b) report the medical evidence regarding the effectiveness of the test. Recommendations for various screening tests are given for both adults and children. Reading through a few of these recommendations can be instructive. If you are not yet familiar with these summaries, visit their methods and processes site (http://www.uspreventiveservicestaskforce.org/methods.htm). You might also want to explore how screening tests are evaluated by the Canadian Task Force on Preventive Health Care (http://canadiantaskforce.ca/).

Designs for Health Policies

There are instances in which the intervention is a health policy, action, or initiative that when implemented affects the health of populations. Almost all such public policies do not involve randomization (the Oregon Experiment is a notable exception) but some, by virtue of where the laws and regulations are enacted, may constitute natural experiments. It may be a regulation regarding vaccination in school children at the state level, or policies regarding health insurance, regulation of tobacco and alcohol sales, regulation of providers, medication regulations, and other policies at the local, regional or national level. Sometimes international comparisons can be very informative as well.

Investigations of populations require the use of population-based electronic databases. A central list of databases in the United States is the Directory of Health and Human Services Data Resources available at the Department of Health and Human Services (http://aspe.hhs.gov/datacncl/DataDir/index.shtml). This list of databases is quite broad and the types of data available for research purposes are dependent upon the particular survey and data source. This is a good place to start because the links to each website are given.

Debate
There have been several studies of screening tests that, when published, were quite controversial. Perhaps you heard about these studies on the news, such as mammograms for breast cancer or prostate-specific antigen (PSA) test for prostate cancer. Choose one of these tests. Find one of the controversial research studies (example: http://www.ncbi.nlm.nih.gov/pubmed/23171096). Often there are arguments to be made on either side of such issues. Debate the evidence for and against use of a specific screening test for people with a low-risk profile and people with a high-risk profile.

Explore
Study designs in health policy and health services research are varied. Go to the *Milbank Quarterly* (http://www.milbank.org/publications/the-milbank-quarterly) and look at the Current Issue. Explore the variety of articles retrieved. Also visit *Health Affairs* (http://www.healthaffairs.org/) and look at the latest issue (Current Issue, top right). Read a few of the abstracts. Anything interesting? Then visit *Medical Care* (http://journals.lww.com/lww-medicalcare/pages/default.aspx) and read through the abstracts of a few original articles and brief reports. Learn something new?

Studies regarding health policies extensively utilize electronic databases and vary in design. One of the natural choices is the interrupted time series with comparators, also known as the controlled time trend analysis design. This can be used to measure pre- versus post-policy changes in outcomes and, when available, include comparators. The comparators may be outcomes in other regions in which the policy did not occur or a different defined policy that was enacted at other locations.

Other appealing options include longitudinal designs such as the cohort study or panel study. Cohort studies would involve observing a defined group of people in the database who have differing experiences because of variations in policy. For example, Medicare provided coverage for glaucoma screening in beneficiaries who have diabetes, a family history of glaucoma, African-Americans aged 50 or older, and Hispanics aged 65 or older. These groups could collectively be considered an "at risk" cohort and followed together. Or each subgroup could form a cohort and be observed over time. The investigator has a choice to compare outcomes across each of these cohorts or to use other beneficiaries as comparators.

For a panel study, the structure of the data and the mechanism of collection determine whether the electronic database could be analyzed via this particular design. When data are collected repeatedly at regular intervals, a panel study could be considered. Another requirement is that the data cover several regions or types of individuals such that there is variation in policy among the participants. The investigator may have the opportunity to assess time-relevant pre- versus post-policy changes in outcome rates and to compare people who are affected by different policies due to peoples' places of residency or their personal characteristics. There may also be instances in which the comparators are not defined by region but rather by workplace, school, or other defining entities in which an initiative occurred in one place but not in another.

Decision modeling may also be employed for analysis of the effects of health policies. This umbrella term includes methods such as decision trees, Markov modeling, Monte Carlo simulation, discrete event simulation, microsimulation, and dynamic modeling. These methods involve the input of data generally from multiple sources. Often surveys from the National Center for Health Statistics can provide needed information or data sources that are listed in the Directory of Health and Human Services Data Resources site (http://aspe.hhs.gov/datacncl/DataDir/index.shtml). There is also a Health and Medical Care Archive, which is the Data Archive of the Robert Wood Johnson Foundation (http://www.icpsr.umich.edu/icpsrweb/content/HMCA/about.html) and is housed at the University of Michigan. It is easily searchable by topic. At the WHO site, the Global Health Observatory is also available, which enables access to more than 50 databases (http://apps.who.int/gho/data/view.main). The World Health Organization/Europe portal to health statistics also can provide data sources for health policy (http://www.euro.who.int/en/what-we-do/data-and-evidence/databases). Sometimes health statistics are readily available through tools online and can be directly used within the decision models of interest.

Considerations with Large Databases

There is increasing availability of electronic integrated databases for health-related research. In some countries, such as Denmark, all primary care physicians use electronic medical records and nearly all primary care practices have full electronic clinical functioning capabilities (Protti, 2010). Patients see their laboratory results online, as well as their hospital and clinic discharge abstracts. This embracement of technology has led to some important research studies in the medical literature.

While the availability of electronic data has presented opportunities for research that can yield evidence relevant for decision making, aspects of the database that are important to consider prior to a research study include the following:

- ¤ **Longitudinal structure and capabilities of the underlying data.** Think of this issue in terms of the objectives of comparative effectiveness research. Investigators would like to find out whether various therapies impact outcomes in patients. At its core, this requires that the therapies should precede the outcome, and therefore one needs underlying longitudinal data to scientifically prove this. Dates would be best—or at least the time between initiation of a therapy and the outcomes. From a programming point of view, dates are useful because you can calculate the time between dates for many of the variables. Therefore, investigate the underlying structure of the data in the large data warehouses. If a certain database is built only on cross-sectional data with no information regarding time and direct patient-response to a therapy, this may be useful for certain health applications but is less useful in comparative effectiveness research.
- ¤ **Types of services provided.** Data warehouses often originate around a certain group of people, such as patients within a network of hospitals or individuals covered by a certain health insurance policy. Do the underlying data represent only a small slice of a person's life,

---

Take A Look

Go to PubMed (http://www.ncbi.nlm.nih.gov/pubmed) and search for Denmark million. Look at the number of research studies published from Denmark using millions of participants. For example, in an article on stroke after herpes zoster, the Danish investigators used 4.6 million people with 52.9 million person-years of follow-up. Wow. A different article on birthweight and leukemia risk in parents utilized 2.4 million parents of 2 million children. The researchers did not find that birthweight was associated with leukemia risk, but they surely had sufficient power to detect this association if there were one! A benefit of complete electronic coverage of populations is the ability to investigate rare diseases. The investigators using the Danish population have the capabilities of examining exposures (and therefore, possible preventive strategies) and complications associated with rare diseases.

Another advantage of complete electronic coverage of populations is the ability to achieve one of the core objectives of comparative effectiveness research— that is, to provide results in enough detail so that subgroups of people can be evaluated. This allows the investigators to give patients meaningful results. Take a look at some of the details available from a study of seizures after vaccination (http://jama.jamanetwork.com/article.aspx?articleid=1355993). Look at the results regarding stratification by gender, timing, and number of vaccinations. Do you think this information may be useful when discussing the benefits and risks of vaccination with parents of young children?

---

such as what occurred during a single hospitalization? Is information regarding other medical services, such as their outpatient visits and other relevant personal characteristics, unavailable? Examine the database closely and inquire regarding how this database was constructed and the types of information it contains. Keep any restrictions in mind when you consider whether your area of interest regarding the effectiveness of certain therapies would be adequately captured in the database.

- **Level of detail regarding outcomes**. It is not uncommon for large health care databases to contain information regarding diagnoses and mortality. It is less common to see detailed information such as how walking ability improved over a specific time period or how feelings of anxiety decreased after certain treatments. Patient-reported outcomes are uncommon in many large databases. Self-reports of mental and physical changes over time in response to various factors are not frequently captured, although there is an intent to include such information more routinely with comparative effectiveness research. If such variables are not available in existing databases and they are essential to the hypothesis, you may need to consider an original research design.

- **The opportunity for discovery**. Sometimes data from linked sources can provide a rich combination of information that, in totality, has not yet been evaluated. Take an outcome such as hospital admission. Being in the hospital is risky in itself, above and beyond the reason for admission. You could catch an infection, or you may not be able to get a good night's sleep. Moreover, a hospital stay may have unanticipated lingering effects after discharge. Imagine that you have access to a rich source of linked databases that contains information regarding what was occurring in peoples' lives in the year before their hospitalization. You have information regarding all their visits to health care practitioners—doctors, therapists, dentists, optometrists—and the medications and therapies they were given. You also have information regarding their mental and physical functioning over time, as well as data regarding their social networks (e.g., whether they live alone, the number of children who live nearby). What a treasure of information to use to try to explain and predict why some people end up hospitalized! This then provides an opportunity to maximize the totality of this information to discover the forces that drive hospital admission.

Discuss

Complex modeling with information from large databases has the potential for providing new insights into health care. Debate the benefits and risks of using complex modeling and data mining for comparative effectiveness research. When preparing for the debate, look at some examples of data integration for decision making in health care such as the Archimedes Model (http://archimedesmodel.com/) and several of the IBM Watson applications within health care (http://www-03.ibm.com/innovation/us/watson/).

If you have the opportunity to use large databases that contain thousands of variables, it may be tempting to go straight to the analysis phase. The variables are right in front of you; just build the mathematical equations and start analyzing. There are pitfalls associated with not defining a good research question, not clarifying the study groups, not thinking about the comparators and outcomes in context, and not looking at the time relationships among factors of interest. With no steering mechanisms, it would be difficult to model relationships in the context of real life.

Dealing with Potential Bias and Confounding: A fair head-to-head comparison in comparative effectiveness research is important. If the participants in the comparison groups are systematically different because of how they were selected (selection bias) or how the measures were observed during the study (information bias), this may pose a problem. **Selection bias** is reduced in trials through concealed randomization. **Information bias** can be reduced in studies through accurate and reliable measurement of the study variables. There is another issue, however, that can occur in observational studies that may affect a fair head-to-head comparison of therapies. This problem is **confounding** by extraneous third variables that are (a) associated with the outcome, (b) associated with the comparators, and (c) not within the underlying causal pathway. There are analytical methods available that can be utilized to abate potential confounding. Some of these approaches are:

- **Multivariable adjustment.** This approach, using typical frequentist statistics, is frequently used in the medical literature. Regression models may include potential confounders as covariates when evaluating the association between comparator choices and the outcome. While patient characteristics and other measured factors in the study can be included in such models, the effects of unknown confounders (if present) are still not addressed.
- **Propensity analyses.** In this approach, the conditional probability of each subject belonging to the intervention group (often baseline patient characteristics) is used to develop a propensity score to account for the effects of such potential confounding factors. There are several related approaches, one in which propensity scores are added to a conventional regression model and another involving propensity matching of subjects through design and analyses. Similar to multivariable adjustment, propensity analyses deals with confounders that were measured within the study and do not address unknown confounders.
- **Instrumental variable.** An instrumental variable is an entity that is related to an explanatory variable (in this instance, the comparators or therapies) and is *only* related to the outcome through this explanatory variable. Methods using instrumental variables can be used to abate

the effects of potential confounders, noncompliance, or measurement error. Instrumental variables have the potential to address confounding by measured and unmeasured variables, but such variables have been difficult to find for many hypotheses. Examples of instruments that have been used in medical research include the geographical distance from services for treatment and preference patterns in drug prescriptions.

Strategies for Selecting the Design

There are general principles and tactics that a researcher can utilize in order to reach a decision regarding study design. When considering various approaches, keep an open mind and discuss options with colleagues. Here are a few strategic suggestions:

1. **The Contrast Approach.** Declare the research question or hypothesis in detail. Make a large grid using the possible study designs on one axis and potential advantages of specific designs along the other axis (e.g., ability to include patient-reported outcomes, ability to report findings by specific patient subgroups). Fill in the grid with your colleagues. Brainstorm how one would design a study to answer this particular research question within each of the study designs. Compare advantages and disadvantages of each design. Are there some designs that could not answer the research question and therefore can be eliminated? Ask experienced practitioners and investigators when issues arise.

2. **The Ranked Approach.** Start with the most rigorous study designs—trials with randomization and trials with within-person comparisons. Consider the feasibility of the most rigorous designs first for your particular research question or hypothesis. If the most rigorous study designs are not feasible or ethical, then work your way down to other, less rigorous designs that may be feasible. Randomization is considered to be one of the most crucial elements of scientific rigor, although randomization of few individuals may not provide balance in the study arms. Another rigorous design is the within-person comparison, although it is only appropriate for specific types of hypotheses. Other elements of scientific rigor include blinding (of either the comparators and/or assessment of the outcomes) and the ability to use an entire population (or random sample or representative sample of the population) rather than a convenience sample of a selected group. There have been published lists of general rankings yielding orders such as randomized controlled

trial, nonrandomized trial, prospective cohort study, retrospective cohort study, and case-control study. Yet, in comparative effectiveness research, this general ranking does not approach the detail necessary for all the options available. One of the ways to start this process is to first ask yourself, "If I were to design the most perfect study for this particular hypothesis, what would it look like?" Forget about feasibility for the moment. Just think about perfection. Brainstorm this question with colleagues. Then, after the ideal is delineated, start looking at the details and which elements that you could not possibly incorporate.

3. **The Upshot Method.** Take a few minutes to imagine that you are a journalist and that your study was just published. You are trying to explain, in a nutshell, the upshot of your study. What did you find? Think deeply about the metric you would use to explain your study in an understandable way to the general public. Look at the outcome in your research question and imagine what would be its most important element. Consider a study in which children who used therapy A had, on average, six fewer seizures each month than children who used therapy B. That metric, six fewer seizures per month, is a mean difference in frequency between A and B. Think about how this outcome could be captured; you would most likely record the frequency of seizures prospectively over time (at least one month and perhaps many months). This requires longitudinal data. Trials are prospective, and so are prospective cohort studies. Start from there and consider the possibilities of such approaches for your particular research question. After you have considered your primary metric of importance, then include any secondary metrics of importance. Structure your design to achieve these goals. This approach works from a consideration of the back end of the study—I know what I want and how do I get there? This particular tactic may require a bit of experience, but occasionally it may be self-evident which study designs are preferable.

4. **The Gap Method.** With this approach, the investigator examines the existing evidence including systematic reviews and meta-analyses already conducted on a particular hypothesis. Occasionally you may find that there is a gap in the evidence—some unknown aspect of the effects of therapies on outcomes. Sometimes this gap is due to a flaw that has not been overcome in the previous research. For example, suppose that the comparators relate to the quantity of platelets utilized for specific patients. If a researcher compares outcomes in groups of patients given different quantities of platelets, are we sure that it is the quantity of platelets that drives the outcome, or is it the underlying reason the platelets were given in the first place (e.g., loss of blood,

inability to produce sufficient numbers of platelets) that drives the outcome? This is called confounding by indication. The platelets were indicated for such patients. A fix for confounding by indication is to conduct a randomized trial with different comparators. The investigator starts with all patients in whom platelets are indicated and then randomizes to treatment choices (different dosages). Then you have separated out indication from true treatment effects. In general, the gap method starts with a review of the existing literature with a subsequent assessment of problems with the current evidence. The investigator finds a design that will rectify these problems.

For researchers considering various design approaches prior to the start of the study, there are mechanisms available to help with group discussions among the collaborators. For example, there is a Pragmatic-Explanatory Continuum Indicator Summary instrument, which has been successfully used when designing randomized trials (Thorpe, 2009). It is a graphic instrument that looks like a wheel or spider web in which researchers assess flexibilities and degrees of intensity for various study features, or domains such as intensity of follow-up of trial participants (http://www.cmaj.ca/content/180/10/E47.full). When discussing the different options one should keep in mind certain aspects of comparative effectiveness research, including choosing viable comparators and applying them in real-world settings, more comprehensive inclusion of patients, and the use of patient-reported outcomes or outcomes that have direct relevance to patients and clinicians.

Think
Can you think of other ways to help choose one study design over another? Try thinking of a few additional considerations that may be useful. Also keep in mind that sometimes there are new designs proposed in the literature and that methodology science is not stagnant. If your comparators or outcomes are a bit unusual, brainstorm about how you can fit your particular question into a suitable design. You might use a slight variation of an existing design.

It is also important to remember that patients (and their families/caregivers) who have experience with specific diseases or conditions may be a great resource of knowledge regarding practical measures to consider when designing a study and for insight regarding relevant outcomes. Seek such opinions when possible. Sometimes pilot studies or focus groups may be informative.

Guidance from agencies that provide oversight for clinical research in humans can be useful when selecting specific design features. The Center for Medical Technology Policy (http://www.cmtpnet.org/) distributed recommendations for the conduct of pragmatic clinical trials. These were housed in an effectiveness guidance document (http://cmtpnet.org/wp-content/uploads/downloads/2011/09/PCT3EGD.pdf).

The Perfect Fit

A well-designed study can provide important information that may change the course of peoples' lives. The investigative team and their design decisions are instrumental in making this happen. Yet keep one truism in mind: *There is no single perfect study*. (If you ever find one, let me know!) All studies have advantages and disadvantages. In medicine and science in general, knowledge is gained through the compilation of evidence from a body of studies over time and across disciplines, including both basic sciences and clinical disciplines. Given that a single study cannot achieve perfection, investigators should keep in mind that planning a study involves recognizing, evaluating, and weighing the options available. Wise choices by investigators will yield good studies and enhance our abilities to answer meaningful questions.

10

The Plan

If this is your first adventure into research, the process can seem a bit daunting at first. Yet it is quite feasible if you divide it into stages, step by step. Since comparative effectiveness research involves different types of designs, there is no definitive rigid approach. However, there are some general elements that are part of the process. Below is a simplification of the process, but should provide some overall perspective. The general steps in conducting comparative effectiveness research are:

- **Begin with an idea.** Develop the research questions and hypotheses. Review current state of knowledge. Decide the specific aims and overall objective of the project.
- **Decide on the design and write the research strategy.** Consider design options. Write up the study protocol to include details regarding the design features, the participants in the study, the definitions of the comparators, and the definitions of the patient-centered outcomes, setting, and timing.
- **Apply for funding.** Submit your research strategy to potential funders. Funding for preliminary or pilot studies may be sought first. Larger studies with preliminary data may be submitted later. (Some researchers suggest that funders should be approached first, when beginning your idea. This will give you a clue as to which areas are of greater interest to your potential funders.)
- **Obtain human subjects approval.** While waiting to hear whether your proposal is to be funded, you can submit all the paperwork necessary for human subjects approval at your institution.
- **Obtain the necessary permissions and regulatory agreements.** If funding and human subjects approval are obtained, sometimes there are other approvals that are required. For example, a data use agreement is necessary before obtaining data from the Centers for Medicare and Medicaid Services.
- **Register the trial.** If your study is a trial, register it within one of the standard trial registries (see below). Registries are now being developed for the voluntary registration of other study designs.

- **Develop the study protocol.** Before starting the investigation, develop a detailed plan for implementation. The study protocol should provide direction for all the investigators and ancillary personnel who work within the study. Often an electronic tracking database is initiated, creating the variables necessary so that the participants can be monitored. If Web-based entry of other study aspects is required, these systems should be put in place.
- **Implement the study.** Implementation should follow the study protocol. For prospective studies, enrollment of subjects would commence. For randomized trials, concealed randomization is conducted accordingly to protocol. Interventions are administered and outcomes recorded per protocol. For studies utilizing retrospective databases, this phase generally consists of the computer programming necessary to set up the files prior to analysis.
- **Analyze the data.** The quality of the data is assessed first. This is followed by the analytical procedures as indicated in the protocol.
- **Disseminate the results.** There may be several presentations at scientific conferences and journal publications from a single study, so plan on how and when each will be conducted.
- **Integrate the results into practice.** This may involve several approaches to informing consumers and providers regarding how these results inform decision making. Sometimes the evidence is used to develop clinical guidelines. The integration itself may form the foundation for a different comparative effectiveness research study, such as developing a patient decision aid and assessing its effects on decision-making and outcomes.

These are broad steps, and there is depth into each of these aspects. Depending upon the research question and the design (prospective versus retrospective), there may be alterations to the sequence and content of this general approach. Basically, it is the implementation of a thoughtful plan. There are instances in which it may be useful to begin with a pilot study first and then move on to a larger, more complex study. If you fortunate to be a part of or affiliated with an existing study, tag along with the experienced researchers and learn by watching what they do throughout the project.

Human Subjects

All studies using human subjects need to undergo human subjects review. Institutional Review Boards (IRBs) are entities that provide oversight of studies using humans. They are committees that review, approve (or disapprove), and monitor human studies. All comparative effectiveness research should undergo human subjects review or undergo an evaluation for exemption. Even in instances in which the data are in public use and the information is de-identified, you should apply for an exemption for review. This process involves describing your study to the board and the reasons why it should be exempted. For those projects submitted for full IRB review, information should be provided regarding the objectives, design, protocol, and any aspects of the study that would involve the basic rights of human subjects. Research institutions have standing committees, protocols, and defined procedures for completing the forms necessary for review.

The guiding principles for the protection of human subjects during research are similar, but vary slightly from country to country. In the United States, the Belmont Report delineates three basic ethical principles:

1. **Respect for persons**. This maintains that people should enter into research voluntarily, with the necessary information to make this choice. Such voluntary informed consent involves giving sufficient information regarding the study (purpose, procedures, risks, benefits, alternatives) and allowing the person a chance to ask questions, including giving specific contact information if he or she has further questions at a later time. It also requires that each person be told that they may drop out of the study at any time regardless of reason. There are certain regulations for people who cannot voluntarily provide informed consent because of age (children), cognitive and mental abilities, and for vulnerable persons such as prisoners.
2. **Beneficence**. Beneficence involves an evaluation of the risks and the benefits of participating in the study. Such risks and benefits should be clearly stated and the probability and magnitude of such risks and benefits should be evaluated and defined. Risks should be minimized, as well as methods to achieve the study goal. Brutal or inhumane treatment is never justified.
3. **Justice**. Justice involves the fair and just selection of people for a study. People should not be selected based on unjust reasons—either by favor or by disdain. People should be selected in such a way as to prevent unfair discrimination by social, racial, sexual, or cultural biases.

You might ask yourself why many people participate in research studies after being informed of all the risks and procedures. I have been pleasantly surprised at the level of interest in research by patients and individuals not within the health professions. Clear explanations help. Giving the individual time to ask any questions is important. Informing individuals that they have the right to withdraw from a study at any time (for any reason) can be very comforting. If they don't want to do it anymore, they don't have to. This stipulation can provide relief and shows respect for their decisions.

The World Health Organization provides templates of human consent forms for various types of clinical studies (http://www.who.int/rpc/research_ethics/informed_consent/en/) and they are available for inspection and use. If you work at an educational institution, institute, or company that usually conducts human research, your institution probably has at least one Institutional Review Board, and you can obtain examples or templates of consent forms from them. Keep in mind that such forms are mandatory if your Institutional Review Board stipulates that informed consent is necessary in your study.

Ethical principles in human subjects research are also described in the Declaration of Helsinski, which is available from the World Medical Association and freely available for downloading online (http://www.wma.net/en/30publications/10policies/b3/). In addition, guidelines for human subjects research are provided by the Council for International Organizations of Medical Sciences (http://www.cioms.ch/index.php/bioethics). This international nongovernmental agency provides information regarding ethics in human studies. The International Compilation of Human Research Standards is a good central source (http://www.hhs.gov/ohrp/international/intlcompilation/intlcompilation.html) which contains topic-relevant links. It provides a fairly comprehensive list of key organizations, legislation, regulations, and guidelines for human studies.

Registering a Trial

The International Committee of Medical Journal Editors (http://www.icmje.org/) requires that researchers must register their human trials as a prerequisite for publication in member journals. Trial registration should occur before enrollment of the first subject. Therefore, as soon as you receive funding for the trial and your protocol is set in place, register your trial before you enroll the first participant.

The International Committee of Medical Journal Editors accepts registration in the following registries: ClinicalTrials.gov, Australian New Zealand Clinical Trials Registry (www.anzctr.org.au), the International Standard Randomised Controlled Trial Number Register (http://www.isrctn.org/) also known as ISRCTN, University hospital

Think
People are often concerned about personal privacy when discussing computer records of their health information. First, see if you can find what types of variables constitute Protected Health Information or PHI. Do you have any of your own PHI freely available on the Web? US federal privacy rules related to health data can be found at this site: http://www.hhs.gov/ocr/privacy/hipaa/understanding/summary/index.html. Look at the information regarding what is protected, general principles, and permitted uses. Can you make a list of at least 10 different ways in which you could protect the privacy of electronic health records when conducting a research study?

> **Explore**
> Go to ClinicalTrials.gov (http://clinicaltrials.gov/) or the WHO International Clinical Trials Registry Platform (http://apps.who.int/trialsearch/). Search for whatever topic is of interest to you. Look at the types of information that are displayed. Examine the directions for registering a trial. At the ClinicalTrials site, you can register directly. At the WHO site, you need to first go to the website of one of the primary registries.

Medical Information Network Clinical Trial Registry from Japan (http://www.umin.ac.jp/ctr/index.htm), The Netherlands National Trial Register (http://www.trialregister.nl/trialreg/index.asp), the Community Clinical Trial System also known as EudraCT (https://eudract.ema.europa.eu/), and primary registries that participate in the WHO International Clinical Trials Registry Platform or ICTRP (http://www.who.int/ictrp/network/primary/en/index.html).

Guidelines for Comparative Effectiveness Research

There are guidelines to assist with both the planning and reporting of comparative effectiveness research. In fact, there multiple guidelines with various acronyms—so many that it can set your head spinning (GRADE, GRACE, PRISMA, MOOSE, AMSTAR, CONSORT, QUADAS, etc.). Let's begin with some guidelines that speak directly to comparative effectiveness research. Many of these are used to evaluate research that has already been conducted, but such guidelines can be very instructive in the planning stages as well. Read these guidelines prior to starting your study. Don't wait until your study is finished and then discover that perhaps you should have done something a bit differently. Know what you are getting into from the beginning. Reading these guidelines can help you develop more rigorous and valid studies.

GRADE

Grading of Recommendations Assessment, Development, and Evaluation (GRADE) is a method by which the totality of evidence regarding a particular clinical question can be evaluated. The GRADE approach is used worldwide and was intended to unify the various evidence-based approaches into a common approach for evaluating medical evidence. It utilizes a comprehensive method to appraise the entire body of studies conducted on a topic. The approach is systematic and transparent. The evidence is graded from high to moderate, low, and very low. The factors within the scoring system include the type of evidence (study design), the quality of the study based on study-specific features, consistency of the effect, directness (generalizability), and effect size. The final GRADE score varies from high (four or more points) to very low (one point or less) describing the quality of the evidence for a specific intervention and its specific outcome or effect. Well-conducted randomized controlled trials are given high quality evidence. GRADE is used for summary activities such as for writing systematic reviews and for developing clinical guidelines.

The criteria used by GRADE to assign levels of evidence are as follows:

- Type of evidence:
  - Randomized trial = high
  - Observational study = low
  - Any other evidence = very low
- Decrease grade if:
  - Serious or very serious limitation to study quality
  - Important inconsistency
  - Some or major uncertainty about directness
  - Imprecise or sparse data
  - High probability of reporting bias
- Increase grade if:
  - Strong evidence of association—significant relative risk of > 2 (< 0.5) based on consistent evidence from 2 or more observational studies, with no plausible confounders (+1)
  - Very strong evidence of association—significant relative risk of > 5 (< 0.2) based on direct evidence with no major threats to validity (+2)
  - Evidence of a dose response gradient (+1)
  - All plausible confounders would have reduced the effect (+1) or would suggest a spurious effect when results show no effect (+1)

The final Summary of Findings table lists the quality of the evidence in an understandable format, with the circles with plus signs indicating strength and the empty circles indicating lower quality of evidence. The range of evidence is categorized as follows:

- High quality evidence ⊕⊕⊕⊕
- Moderate quality evidence ⊕⊕⊕○
- Low quality evidence ⊕⊕○○
- Very low quality evidence ⊕○○○

PRISMA

The Preferred Reporting Items for Systematic Reviews and Meta-Analyses (PRISMA) statement is a set of recommendations for researchers who wish to report a systematic review or meta-analysis of randomized trials. It currently includes a 27-item checklist and a four-phase flow diagram. Although

Explore
The GRADE Working Group (http://www.gradeworkinggroup.org/) and McMaster University (http://cebgrade.mcmaster.ca/) have readily available information regarding GRADE and links. Examples of the Summary of Findings tables are given. Look at some of the types of investigations that utilized the GRADE method (select Publications tab on the GRADE Working Group site). You can also download their GRADEpro software and try it out. GRADE is also on Facebook and Twitter.

> **Take A Look**
> The PRISMA statement and checklist are openly available online (http://www.prisma-statement.org/). Find the checklist available in tabular format and the flow diagram. Occasionally there are updates, so if you are conducting a systematic review or meta-analysis, check back to see if there have been any revisions. Go also to the main JAMA site online (http://jama.jamanetwork.com/journal.aspx) and type in PRISMA in the search box. Explore the different meta-analyses that utilized the PRISMA statement in their methods.

the guidelines are meant for reporting of the research at the end of the study, the researcher would be wise to look through these when designing the study so that the design elements can be incorporated into the study from the start. For example, one of the guidelines on the checklist says, "Present full electronic search strategy for at least one database, including any limits used, such that it could be repeated." This informs the researcher that accurate records should be kept regarding which search terms were used during extraction of the study articles.

MOOSE

Just as the PRISMA statement is generally used to guide the reporting of systematic reviews and meta-analyses from trials, the Meta-Analysis of Observational Studies in Epidemiology (MOOSE) statement is used to guide the reporting of similar studies from observational data. These were published in the *Journal of the American Medical Association* and are openly available online (http://jama.jamanetwork.com/article.aspx?articleid=192614). The statement includes a set of guidelines and checklist on how to report meta-analyses of observational studies such as cohort or case-control studies.

CONSORT

It is important to be aware that there are guidelines for reporting and publication of randomized trials. These are called the Consolidated Standards of Reporting Trials, or CONSORT for short (http://www.consort-statement.org/). The CONSORT statement was originally developed to improve the reporting of parallel randomized trials with two arms, although the guidelines are currently applicable to many types of trials. For researchers, the checklist and the flow diagram are very useful. The checklist currently lists 25 items that relate to how information is presented in the title, abstract, introduction, methods, results, and discussion sections of a typical article. Major medical journals require that authors conform to the CONSORT structure when publishing their results from randomized trials. Over time, various extensions to the CONSORT statement have been developed. For example, design extensions include cluster trials, noninferiority and equivalence trials, and pragmatic trials. Since comparative effectiveness trials, by definition, measure effectiveness in a real-world setting, you should read over the pragmatic trial extension. An example of one of the extensions for pragmatic trials is that the eligibility criteria should include the degree to which the participants and setting reflect everyday practice which, when relevant, include descriptions of the practitioners (e.g., nurses), institutions (e.g., hospitals), and communities or settings. There are also extensions for certain types of interventions, such as non-pharmacological treatment interventions. Data extensions to CONSORT are also available and include patient-reported outcomes. For example, for patient-reported outcomes in a trial, information should be included regarding the instrument used to obtain the outcome (e.g., include the name of the standardized questionnaire), its validity and reliability, and the mechanisms utilized to obtain this information (paper, phone, electronic, etc.).

Check It Out
Go to the CONSORT site and look at the guidelines for each section of a journal article (www.consort-statement.org). Check out the extensive availability of the statements in different medical journals and the information regarding extensions. Are there certain terms listed that you were not yet aware of? A quick way to find articles related to CONSORT is to visit the NICE site (https://www.evidence.nhs.uk/) and type in consort. You can filter by types of information: Primary Research and some of the trials will appear. I just pulled one up on tai chi in patients with heart failure—a single-blind, multisite, parallel-group, randomized controlled trial (http://archinte.jamanetwork.com/article.aspx?articleid=227164). Did the tai chi work better than the educational approach?

SPIRIT

In contrast to CONSORT which serves as a guideline for reporting of trials, Standard Protocol Items: Recommendations for Interventional Trials (SPIRIT) serves as a guideline for trial protocols. That is, the researcher would use the SPIRIT checklist when developing the trial protocol (http://www.spirit-statement.org/). The SPIRIT checklist is currently 33 items and contains additional information regarding the content of such items, rather than the formatting of items. There tends to be overlap between CONSORT and SPIRIT regarding the categories listed, and such guidelines tend to evolve over time; therefore, as a researcher planning a trial, it may be wise to look at both of these checklists when starting your study. If you are a new researcher, reading through the SPIRIT checklist will give you an idea of the types of procedures usually conducted in a randomized trial and can be very informative when writing up the protocol.

Keep in mind that some of these documents are shown in tabular form, indicating that the researcher or staff would fill these out as hard copies. However, most of us complete protocols and develop tracking databases on the computer, so feel free to design your protocol accordingly. You can use the content elements within the SPIRIT checklist as the framework for the variables necessary for input. Make sure that you design a system whereby you and your team can periodically assess progress (e.g., daily, weekly, monthly). Feel free to bring in a programmer experienced in database management for advice, or add him or her to your team.

TREND

The Transparent Reporting of Evaluations with Nonrandomized Designs (TREND) statement was devised to assist with the reporting of nonrandomized controlled trials. There is a 22-item checklist associated with these guidelines that are available at the Centers for Disease Control and Prevention (http://www.cdc.gov/trendstatement/). TREND was designed with public health interventions in mind, in which an intervention would be feasible but randomization would not. For those researchers interested in nonrandomized trials, you might wish to read the statement and follow the checklist during study development and reporting.

> **Take A Look**
> Check out the SPIRIT statement and checklist online (http://www.spirit-statement.org/). Go through the 33-item checklist and look at the types of information considered necessary in each category. A template figure is also downloadable which may be useful when you are developing the protocol. An electronic protocol tool and resource (SEPRe) is anticipated. What other ways could this information be made available in real-time through different communication technologies?

STROBE

The Strengthening the Reporting of Observational studies in Epidemiology (STROBE) statement was developed to improve the reporting of observational studies. There are separate checklists available for cohort studies, case-control studies, cross-sectional studies, and conference abstracts. These checklists are available at: http://www.strobe-statement.org/. If you are planning an observational study, read through the checklist so that all items will be addressed.

GRACE

Good Research for Comparative Effectiveness (GRACE) is an initiative to provide guidelines for observational comparative effectiveness research. Evaluation of studies using the GRACE principles (http://www.graceprinciples.org/index.html) involves questions regarding recording of treatments and outcomes, objectivity and validity of the outcome measurement, consistency of the outcome measurements across treatment groups, accounting for confounders and effect modifiers, initiation of treatment, concurrent comparators, appropriate follow-up and data analyses (Dreyer, 2010).

> **Explore**
> Go to the Grace Principles site (http://www.graceprinciples.org/index.html) and look at their guidelines and checklist in more detail. Also visit the STROBE site (http://www.strobe-statement.org/) to compare how their checklist differs.

OTHER GUIDELINES

There are other guidelines and checklists that are used in medical research. Additional guidelines and statements include the Consolidated Health Economic Evaluation Reporting Standards (CHEERS), Enhancing Transparency in Reporting the Synthesis of Qualitative Research (ENTREQ), Standards for Quality Improvement Reporting Excellence (SQUIRE), Assessment of Multiple Systematic Reviews (AMSTAR), Consolidated Criteria for Reporting Qualitative Research (COREQ), Quality Assessment of Diagnostic Accuracy Studies (QUADAS), and Standards for the Reporting of Diagnostic Accuracy Studies (STARD). There are even systematic reviews of the guidelines. These guidelines tend to change over time, so you must be a bit vigilant regarding changes and new guidelines as they emerge.

> **Explore**
>
> The Equator Network is a good central source for researchers (http://www.equator-network.org/home/). It houses reporting guidelines, author guidelines, editor guidelines, and developer guidelines at one site. This network serves an important function in promoting better reporting, reviewing and editing of health research. As an umbrella organization, they provide cross-disciplinary information with a common purpose: transparent and accurate reporting of health research studies. Explore their site.

Data Management in Clinical Research

In practical terms, there are several general areas pertaining to data management that are important in maintaining adherence to study protocol in comparative effectiveness research studies:

- **Data entry and management**. In clinical studies, secure data entry is necessary to collect information regarding subject characteristics and other information relevant to the study. It is imperative to delineate a protocol for this process and to streamline if possible. If there are several sites involved, it is important to provide a secure network with adherence to all human subject protections. Often one central site is assigned the task of data management. There are several purposes of data collection in most clinical studies:
  - **Data for purposes of enrollment, follow-up and adherence to protocol**. Personal information for each subject may be necessary for contact purposes during clinical studies. Demographic information and other baseline data relevant to the study are collected. Data regarding when the subjects enrolled, when therapy began, adherence to therapies, contact information relevant to study processes, monitoring of outcomes, and other relevant study-specific information are entered. Relational databases for monitoring adherence to protocol are sometimes called tracking files and tend to be fluid, in that new people are entering over time, some of the contact information may change, some subjects may drop out, and so forth. The intent of such files is smooth implementation during the time course of the study. Routine reports are generated regarding how well the enrollment, administration of therapies, and measurement of outcomes

are progressing during the study. Increasingly, there are openly available management tools that assist with data-related aspects of clinical research. One tool is REDCap (http://catalyst.harvard.edu/services/redcap/), and another is OpenClinica (https://community.openclinica.com/).

- **Data for purposes of analysis of study hypotheses.** Analysis files or databases include the variables to be utilized in analyses to answer the specific research questions. Often personal data such as names or addresses are excluded. Variables regarding subject characteristics, comparators, and outcomes are included. Data capture for this main statistical database is critical for the reporting of final results, and quality checks should be incorporated into the study to assess accuracy. Often programming must be done to structure the variables in the necessary constructs and formats for analyses. Sometimes the information comes from linking a number of different sources, and the programmer generates new variables that are necessary so that the analyses can proceed.
- **Data analyses.** There is no one analytic approach that is performed for all types of comparative effectiveness research. Procedures depend upon the *a priori* hypothesis, the structure of the design, and the mathematical properties of the measures being assessed. Details regarding how to choose and perform specific types of analyses are available. There are stand-alone courses and textbooks on specific statistical procedures. You are urged to explore. As a researcher, you will either perform these procedures yourself or work with others with this knowledge. In either instance, you will be required to interpret the results of studies and this involves knowledge of what these statistics mean.

Incorporation of Evidence into Practice and Everyday Life

STAGES OF IMPLEMENTATION

When the relative effectiveness of a therapy has been demonstrated, the next step is to implement these findings into clinical practice and our everyday lives. This is a very important element that does not necessarily occur without mechanisms in place to foster these changes. The National Implementation Research Network (http://nirn.fpg.unc.edu/) has identified several stages that occur during the process of implementation of therapies in practice:

- **Exploration stage.** During this stage there is a consideration of the needs of the patients or individuals involved, the fit with current

practices and values, the availability of resources, an expectation of outcomes if the therapy were implemented, readiness for replication in similar settings, and the capacity for implementation.
- **Installation.** During this stage, preparations are made before initiation. Mechanisms are put in place to ensure that the new initiatives or practices are ready to start.
- **Initial implementation.** During this stage, the practice or therapy is first initiated. Starting a new therapy may involve compelling forces associated with the *status quo* and the integration of new practices.
- **Full implementation.** During this stage, the practice is fully operational and integrated into practice. The components of the initiative are being implemented and adaptation occurs. The therapy becomes standard practice.

Some also include a fifth stage called **program sustainability**, in which practices are in place to ensure that the program is maintained over time.

EFFECTIVE METHODS FOR DIFFUSION

Comparative effectiveness research yields information regarding the types of therapies that work best for specific people at a particular time. But if such information lingers in the academic literature without dissemination to patients and providers, the ultimate purpose of comparative effectiveness research will not be met. End user adoption and institutionalization are the final steps within the process of comparative effectiveness research. Some of the more effective methods for diffusing evidence into daily practice involve the following:

- Involvement of mass media in patient education
- Spearheading by practitioner champions
- Expert consultations
- Opinion leaders
- Changes in reimbursement or cost
- Academic detailing (educational outreach to providers)
- Auditing and feedback
- Performance gap assessment
- Preliminary pilot of the new practice or approach

Sometimes such methods are combined with others, such as interactive provider education with one of the approaches given above. In health care settings, feedback mechanisms built into computerized decision support, or prompts with checklists and reminders, also tend to have some effect on practice change. In addition, services not found to be effective through well-conducted research studies may not be reimbursable over time by insurance, and therefore this can influence the frequency of specific practices. Societal forces also play a part. Being a part of a larger social system that embraces the new practices generally is helpful in facilitating change in group members.

There are several ongoing projects to promote communication of comparative effectiveness research and integration into practice. One project, Developing and Evaluating Communication Strategies to Support Informed Decisions and Practices Based on Evidence (DECIDE), was formed to improve the dissemination of evidence-based recommendations by developing and evaluating methods for the dissemination of guidelines (http://www.decide-collaboration.eu/). They develop targeted dissemination strategies for providing information to patients, providers, and other stakeholders, by utilizing recommendations generated from GRADE (Grading of Recommendations Assessment, Development, and Evaluation).

The US Agency for Healthcare Research and Quality sponsors initiatives to integrate comparative effectiveness research into clinical practice and to inform patients regarding therapies and services so to enhance more informed health decision-making. The John M. Eisenberg Center for Clinical Decisions and Communications Science uses medical evidence to produce consumer products such as research summaries and patient decision aids.

Explore
Go to the National Center for Biotechnology Information site on Comparative Effectiveness Review Summary Guides for Clinicians (http://www.ncbi.nlm.nih.gov/books/NBK43420/). Listed are topic-specific guides relevant to practice such as first-generation versus second-generation antipsychotics in adults, comparisons of surgical treatments for open-angle glaucoma, treatments for chronic hepatitis C virus infection, and so forth. Scroll down until you see a topic that is of interest to you and read through the guide. Look at the sections entitled Clinical Bottom Line, Patient-Related Quality of Life, Gaps in Knowledge, What To Discuss With Your Patients and Their Caregivers, Resources, and other topics. Are there certain sections that you think would be particularly important? Do you have any suggestions on ways to improve these sections or to include other sections?

Centers in the United States specifically charged with generating this evidence include the Evidence-based Practice Centers which conduct evidence-based systematic reviews of services and therapies (http://effectivehealthcare.ahrq.gov/index.cfm/who-is-involved-in-the-effective-health-care-program1/about-evidence-based-practice-centers-epcs/). Currently there are 11 Centers which conduct reviews. Centers for Education and Research on Therapeutics (CERTs) conduct research and provide information regarding health information technology, therapies for heart and blood vessel disorders, mental health therapeutics, musculoskeletal disorders, pediatric therapeutics, and tools for optimizing medication safety (http://www.certs.hhs.gov/centers/centers.htm). The Developing Evidence to Inform Decisions about Effectiveness Network is a network of centers and researchers that conduct research regarding comparative clinical effectiveness as well.

There are also dissemination initiatives that are evidence-based and are targeted to specific health conditions. One such site is the National Registry of Evidence-based Programs and Practices (http://www.nrepp.samhsa.gov/). It provides information regarding therapies and interventions that have shown benefit in promoting mental health, preventing substance abuse, and treating mental health-related conditions. Their site includes a quality of research section in which the evidence is rated, and a readiness for dissemination section where the therapies are evaluated for availability criteria.

EDUCATIONAL METHODS WITH PATIENTS AND POPULATIONS

Educators have long known that interaction and engagement facilitate learning. This is true with health education as well. Incorporating evidence-based therapies into everyday practice requires this engagement—for both patients and clinicians. Shared decision making is a renewed effort to create mechanisms in which both patients and their health providers communicate and discuss evidence-based options. This may be a challenge, since there is not yet a great body of scientific research regarding structure, formats, timing, and communication techniques in all medical settings and with particular therapies. Yet the options available are becoming more diverse.

Patient decision aids and consumer-usable sites on evidence-based decision making tend to be known by researchers and health professionals but may not be

Check It Out
The Substance Abuse & Mental Health Services Administration has a website for the National Registry of Evidence-based Programs and Practices (NREPP). Look at their site online (http://www.nrepp.samhsa.gov/). At the top where you can search for an intervention, select the "View All Interventions" tab. Look at the variety of interventions. Go to the bottom of the page and select "Zippy's Friends." Read through the descriptive information and notice that, at the bottom, Quality of Research is available (try selecting it), as well as Readiness for Dissemination, Costs, Replications, and Contact Information. Wow, you can even see costs! Note that a pdf Summary is freely available.
In addition, if you visit their Learning Center (see selection at the very top), one of the choices is Comparative Effectiveness Research. Within their comparative effectiveness research series is a list of selected interventions with booklets, fact sheets, and intervention summaries for practitioners and patients. Take a look at the information for dialectical behavior therapy or eye movement desensitization and reprocessing. Mindfulness-based cognitive therapy also looks interesting, as does motivational interviewing. Check out topics that are of interest to you. This particular educational site is a good illustration of the wise use of health information dissemination.

Try This Out
Go to Mayo Clinic's decision aid on taking aspirin and statins (http://statindecisionaid.mayoclinic.org/). Go ahead and enter the Tool so that you can examine the process. On the top left under Current Risk, put in your characteristics or make up whatever patient profile that you wish. See the diagrammatic representation of your risk of having a heart attack (over the next 10 years). Then select your intervention, either aspirin or statins, or both. Look at your future risk of having a heart attack. You can also see other issues related to this decision regarding cost, daily routine, benefits and risks.

> **Explore**
> Other patient decision aids are available at the Agency for Healthcare Research and Quality (http://effectivehealthcare.ahrq.gov/index.cfm/tools-and-resources/patient-decision-aids/). Select one of the decision aids listed and evaluate how the information is presented, what types of information are given, and the output. A large inventory of patient decision aids is currently available through the Ottawa Hospital Research Institute. Take a look at a list of the decision aids at this site: http://decisionaid.ohri.ca/AZlist.html. Scroll down and see the variety of decision aids available. Let's select "Acne: Should I see my doctor?" In the Decision Aid Summary, there is a section called How to obtain the decision aid. Select the Available here link. Go through the six steps within the decision aid. How does the methodology for this decision aid compare with the others that you have seen?

widely known by the general public. Patient decision aids are tools that help people make decisions relevant to their health. It includes providing evidence-based information and incorporates the patients' values and preferenes.

The Gateway to Health Communication & Social Marketing Practice at the Centers for Disease Control and Prevention is a good starting point for investigators involved in health education (http://www.cdc.gov/healthcommunication/). The materials are of particular relevance for delivery of information to populations. Audience considerations, tools, templates and methods of distribution are discussed. Usability.gov (http://www.usability.gov/) is a resource for creating websites and is worth a look. Note that there are CDC Apps available as well.

For dissemination of general health information, a central hub for evidence-based health information would be useful. Currently in the United States, there are many consumer health sites housed within different federal agencies. MedlinePlus at the National Library of Medicine (http://www.nlm.nih.gov/medlineplus/), Centers for Disease Control and Prevention (http://www.cdc.gov/), healthfinder.gov (http://healthfinder.gov/), Health Information at the National Institutes of Health (http://health.nih.gov/), Patients & Consumers at the Agency for Healthcare Research and Quality (http://www.ahrq.gov), Food and Drug Administration For Consumers site (http://www.fda.gov/ForConsumers/default.htm), the US Department of Agriculture for consumer nutrition (http://www.cnpp.usda.gov/), and many others. For consumers who wish information on particular topics, it may be more functional if the agencies would collaborate to house evidence-based health information through a central hub. It may also be possible in the future to develop global hubs since the relevance of health evidence crosses national borders. It is important to

> **Explore**
> You may be aware of awards given to the top websites each year. One of these awards is called is Webby Awards (http://www.webbyawards.com/index.php). Go to their site and look at some of the Winners (see top link). Explore some of these sites—not necessarily in terms of specific content but how the information was delivered. Look at the visuals and types of interactions available. Can you imagine how some of this creativity may be translated to interactions relevant to health? Keep an open mind. List five different elements that, if you developed your own website, may be candidates for delivering health information or engaging peoples' involvement.

distinguish between health information that is based on the results of scientific studies demonstrating effectiveness (or efficacy) as opposed to the voluminous information regarding health from various media sources which may or may not be evidence-based. Knowledge of study design and comparative effectiveness research should allow greater perception regarding the quality of the health information generally available.

11

THE INSPIRATION

I knew a family. A great family with two wonderful funny parents, three crazy kids, and a big dog. They were always on the go, laughing all the time. One winter day they were off to visit relatives. On a curvy icy road, the accident happened in an instant. Their world turned upside down. Crushed, for one little boy. In an instant, he lost his mother and father, and his older brother. After spending a year in a persistent vegetative state, his little sister passed away as well. His brother and sister had helped to cradle him from the oncoming truck—he was the middle kid sitting in the middle backseat. He is a survivor. An amputee survivor.

In an instant, this little boy entered the world of being a patient: Doctor visits. Rehabilitation. Fitting prostheses. Adapting to a different world and working through mental and physical challenges. Lots of choices and decisions to make. His was a dramatic entry into the world of health care. All of us are a part of that world, though not always thrust into it as this little boy was. Some of us are heavy consumers of health services, and others of us use it just once in a while. I don't shy away from occasionally calling people—even healthy people—patients. It's just a matter of time and opportunity.

You, however, are in a special place because you, as a researcher, have an opportunity to influence lives such as this little boy's. You can test out new models of prostheses against the older models, or participate in studies of limb regeneration. You can design and implement comparative studies, and for all those next little kids (and big kids) who lose a limb, you can improve their lives. You can test out whether there are specific behavioral interventions that help people through challenging periods in their lives. Or you can design studies to test out safety devices that are intended to prevent injuries in the first place.

Welcome to comparative effectiveness research. We need you. For all the patients and families and friends who desire answers, we need your help. This is an area of medical research where everyone is "in," and no one is "out." Everyone plays a part—including us patients. If you are not yet used to conducting or participating in research yet, that's okay. You'll learn. If you are an experienced researcher and clinician, thank you. Help us to engage others to advance our understanding of health and disease.

Exciting Horizons

We are living during exciting times. Our world is becoming more interconnected. Advances in communication and computational sciences are teaming up with developments in functional genomics, nanotechnology, stem cell biology, and a range of interrelated sciences that hold promise for extending healthy life and tackling complex diseases. Scientists from different disciplines who, historically were comfortable within discrete domains, are increasingly crossing boundaries to explore new and creative approaches to solving problems. This widens the opportunities for comparative effectiveness research. The options for comparators are expanding.

Think

In the general media, have you recently heard of any new technologies or methods of communication which could have effects on people's health? Check out some of the latest news on ScienceDaily, EurekAlert!, New Scientist, or other science news outlets. Could any of these approaches possibly be tested as comparators in a research study?

Listed below are a few potential advances on the horizon:

- Electronic devices implanted in the body that dissolve over time.
- Nanotechnology used to create polymer shells around proteins that specifically target cancer cells, but don't harm normal cells.
- Development of synthetic body parts (e.g., trachea, bladder, and other organs).
- XNA (artificial DNA) therapies.
- Electronic brain implant to improve decision making.
- Artificial blood.
- Robotic freedom for persons with limited mobility.
- Bionic eye (retinal implant).
- Graphene biodevices.

Feel free to add to this list, and look for clues as to additional therapies under investigation. Many of these potential treatments could be imagined as a device, drug, or biologic used as a comparator in a trial. Moreover, the expansion of communication technologies opens many avenues for interpersonal collaborations which may have relevance to mental and social health applications.

There are additional recent advances that have particular significance to comparative effectiveness research. The core of this research rests on the decisions that an individual must make regarding choice of therapies. Often the outcomes—be they beneficial or adverse—are not immediate. They may be experienced a month after starting a particular treatment or a year later. Sometimes the wide range of effects may not be seen unless one inspects long trajectories of people's lives. This requires observation over a long period of time or, in other words, a longitudinal database. With the availability of electronic medical records and the linking of large databases, it is possible to examine whether people who made several therapeutic decisions over time have better outcomes than people who made other decisions. So think about this. You have a longitudinal database. It is possible to (retrospectively) travel through time with patients to see what they experienced with the decisions that they made.

This is exactly what some investigators did (Bennett, 2013). They used a large database of patient-level information and applied a computational approach to sequential decision making. They wanted to know whether the database—with all the detailed information—could be used to predict good outcomes for patients. It did. Artificial intelligence did better in deciding which therapies to choose at which times than did practitioners. The computer made better treatment decisions than humans, yielding a 30% to 35% increase in better patient outcomes and saving money to boot. Because there were many treatment decisions, the pathways were complex, and multiple options were available at different points in time, the authors concluded that it may be difficult for humans to process all this information at once. The trajectories were complicated with hundreds of bits of information arising from different aspects of each patient's medical history and current status. The authors suggested that this complex, sequential decision making was better left to computer systems that can process the volume and relationships among data. Clinicians can then be freed to deliver the actual care.

Debate
Does this sound great? Fantastic? Or a bit scary? What are your opinions on computer-assisted decision making? Perhaps you have heard of Watson the IBM computer (which was featured on the TV show "Jeopardy"). It is now being used by providers at various hospitals and clinics, such as the Cleveland Clinic and the Memorial Sloan-Kettering Cancer Center. Will Watson-like systems be the new physician's assistant? See if you can find a few research studies published in which the investigators utilized Watson or another similar system.

The use of evidence-based knowledge derived from a large and diverse body of scientific studies to inform decision-making is at the core of comparative effectiveness research. Clinically relevant databases may shed light on the complex trajectories of life. These examinations may provide insight into what is likely to happen when we take one path—and what could happen if we took another –at critical junctures in our lives. Recommended decisions may be tailored to specific types of people and therefore, in concert with the goals of precision medicine.

One could imagine that these large systems might provide answers to all of our research questions: Just build a grand database and start data mining. But this approach will not adequately answer every research question. It may be very helpful in many respects but, at times, it may be difficult to tease out whether the treatments themselves or the indications for the treatment (i.e., why the treatment was ordered in the first place) were the ultimate drivers of the outcomes. Sometimes there is no substitute for a prospective head-to-head comparison. That's just what investigators did with a study on blood some time ago.

Blood has often been described synonymously with life itself. Blood has historically been viewed as so essential to life that it has been widely transfused in many situations: for patients with injuries, surgical patients, individuals with various types of anemia, patients with blood disorders such as hemophilia, patients with cancer, burn patients, patients with liver disease, and postpartum women. It has been a therapeutic option for at least a century. Since blood has been transfused for many reasons, one might assume that the clinical studies have all been conducted, and the risks and benefits of transfusion have been evaluated in randomized controlled trials. Well, blood is one of those time-honored therapies that had been used in medicine for many years *without* evidence of efficacy from Phase 3 randomized controlled trials. It was thought that such trials—with a "no treatment" or "sham treatment" arm—would be unethical.

But there are ways to conduct such trials that would be ethical. It was a very clever way of devising the intervention. Instead of a "no treatment" arm, the comparison would involve changing the criteria by which a red blood cell transfusion would be ordered. For many years, the standard practice was to transfuse patients whose hemoglobin was 10 g/dL or less or their hematocrit was 30% or less. This was the 10/30 rule: Hold off on the red blood cell transfusions for patients above this level and administer a transfusion if the patient fell below this cut point. These criteria are referred to as transfusion thresholds or triggers. In 1999, the *New England Journal of Medicine* published a randomized controlled trial (http://www.nejm.org/doi/full/10.1056/NEJM199902113400601) conducted by researchers in which critically ill patients were randomized to either a restrictive strategy (transfusion given when hemoglobin <7.0 g/dL) or a liberal strategy (transfusion given when hemoglobin <10.0 g/dL) (Hébert, 1999). One would think that if red blood cell transfusions were therapeutic for critically ill patients, then the patients receiving more transfusions would do better. Not so. They found that the patients receiving the liberal strategy (more transfusions) did not have lower mortality rates than the patients receiving the restrictive strategy (less transfusions). Thirty-day mortality was similar in the two groups. In addition, in patients who were younger and who were less acutely ill, the restrictive strategy (fewer transfusions) resulted in better outcomes. So the results begged the question: If red blood cell transfusions in critically ill patients were not improving their health, are they effective as currently prescribed? This trial, called the TRICC trial or Transfusion Requirements in Critical Care Trial, was an eye-opener. It spawned other trials, and served as a legitimate gateway into investigations of whether red blood cell transfusions are effective in improving the health of specific types of patients. There are currently trials underway to evaluate whether the length of storage of the red blood cells affects outcomes. Sometimes time-honored therapies, when held up for scrutiny, do not achieve the results as expected. So, thank you to the investigators on this project and to the patients who participated. Their work has affected the lives of others.

There are other examples of comparative effectiveness research that originate with a bit of insight. One occurred some time ago in a dentist's office. Going to the dentist is one of those circumstances that may cause some people to cringe: The sound of the drill, the pain. But occasionally, that time spent waiting for the next procedure and looking up at the ceiling takes your mind in different directions. It was during one of these dental visits that a particular patient took great interest in the vibrating ultrasonic device used for cleaning his teeth. The patient began to imagine. His thoughts wondered. But he was no usual dental patient—he happened to be a physician who had been trying to devise a procedure to extract cloudy lenses (cataracts) from patients' eyes. At the time, the current method involved an intensive, invasive procedure with serious complications in patients, resulting in a week or more of bedrest and recovery in the hospital. Lying still for long periods of time in a hospital bed was risky—and sometimes deadly. So this dental patient was imagining whether there was a way to remove a cataract that was less invasive and speeded recovery. Hence his insight regarding ultrasound, after seeing the device used in dentistry. Ultrasound could provide the mechanism to emulsify the cloudy lens so that it can be aspirated (sucked up) and removed. This physician, Dr. Charles Kelman, ultimately invented a procedure known as phacoemulsification for cataract removal. He compared this new technique to other methods (Kelman, 1973), and over the years, perfected this procedure and several others. The results are amazing. Today, a person with a cataract can walk into an outpatient surgical center essentially blind and on the same day, walk out with restored vision. This procedure has helped millions of people throughout the world. It has been particularly beneficial in developing countries for individuals with few resources, where sight is critical for performing everyday tasks. For those who were blind, being able to see again was incredible. That's quality of life! Thanks, Dr. Kelman.

Keeping Your Eyes on the Prize

The prize is health: mental, social, and physical well-being. For those people who are currently healthy, it involves maintaining this health. For those individuals with preexisting conditions, it may be better functioning, improvement of symptoms, or the ability to do activities that are important to you. It may also be the ultimate prize—happiness.

With all the differing approaches to the evaluation of the effectiveness of therapies and services, it is sometimes important to take a moment to refocus on this goal. There are considerable resources—personnel, time, and money—spent on processes that are indirectly related to this goal. Occasionally we must take time to assess the degree to which such goals have been achieved in populations as a whole. Discovering which therapies work, in what types of people, and at what time should lead us in that direction.

It is relatively easy to be a critic, to poke and prod existing medical studies. It is another, quite nobler, task to conduct these studies. We need more good information—actionable intelligence, which comes from well-conducted studies. You, your family, and your friends will have plenty of health-related questions over the course of your lifetimes, the answers to which are yet unknown.

So stick your foot in the water. Try it out. Then plunge in.

BIBLIOGRAPHY

Altman DG, McShane LM, Sauerbrei W, Taube SE. Reporting Recommendations for Tumor Marker Prognostic Studies (REMARK): explanation and elaboration. *PLoS Med.* 2012;9(5):e1001216.

Andrews J, Guyatt G, Oxman AD, et al. GRADE guidelines: 14. Going from evidence to recommendations: the significance and presentation of recommendations. *J Clin Epidemiol.* 2013 Jul;66(7):719–25.

Andrews JC, Schünemann HJ, Oxman AD, et al. GRADE guidelines: 15. Going from evidence to recommendation-determinants of a recommendation's direction and strength. *J Clin Epidemiol.* 2013 Jul;66(7):726–35.

Avorn J, Fischer M. "Bench to behavior": translating comparative effectiveness research into improved clinical practice. *Health Aff (Millwood).* 2010;29(10):1891–900.

Baicker K, Taubman SL, Allen HL, et al.; Oregon Health Study Group, Carlson M, Edlund T, Gallia C, Smith J. The Oregon experiment—effects of Medicaid on clinical outcomes. *N Engl J Med.* 2013 May 2;368(18):1713–22.

Balkrishnan R, Chang J, Patel I, Yang F, Merajver SD. Global comparative healthcare effectiveness research: evaluating sustainable programmes in low & middle resource settings. *Indian J Med Res* 2013;137(3):494–501.

Balshem H, Helfand M, Schünemann HJ, et al. GRADE guidelines: 3. Rating the quality of evidence. *J Clin Epidemiol.* 2011 Apr;64(4):401–06.

Basch E, Abernethy AP, Mullins CD, et el. Recommendations for incorporating patient-reported outcomes into clinical comparative effectiveness research in adult oncology. *J Clin Oncol.* 2012 Dec 1;30(34):4249–55.

Bennett CC, Hauser K. Artificial intelligence framework for simulating clinical decision-making: a Markov decision process approach. *Artif Intell Med.* 2013 Jan;57(1):9–19.

Bossuyt PM, Reitsma JB, Bruns DE, et al; Standards for Reporting of Diagnostic Accuracy. Towards complete and accurate reporting of studies of diagnostic accuracy: the STARD initiative. *Ann Intern Med.* 2003 Jan 7;138(1):40–44.

Boutron I, Moher D, Altman DG, Schulz K, Ravaud P, for the CONSORT group. Methods and processes of the CONSORT group: example of an extension for trials assessing nonpharmacologic treatments. *Ann Intern Med.* 2008 Feb 19;148(4):W60–6.

Brouwers MC, Thabane L, Moher D, Straus SE. Comparative effectiveness research paradigm: implications for systematic reviews and clinical practice guidelines. *J Clin Oncol.* 2012 Dec 1;30(34):4202–07.

Brunetti M, Shemilt I, Pregno S, et al. GRADE guidelines: 10. Considering resource use and rating the quality of economic evidence. *J Clin Epidemiol.* 2013 Feb;66(2):140–50.

Calvert M, Blazeby J, Altman DG, Revicki DA, Moher D, Brundage MD; CONSORT PRO Group. Reporting of patient-reported outcomes in randomized trials: the CONSORT PRO extension. *JAMA.* 2013 Feb 27;309(8):814–22.

Campbell MK, Piaggio G, Elbourne DR, Altman DG; for the CONSORT Group. Consort 2010 statement: extension to cluster randomised trials. *BMJ*. 2012 Sep 4;345:e5661.

Carpenter WR, Meyer AM, Abernethy AP, Stürmer T, Kosorok MR. A framework for understanding cancer comparative effectiveness research data needs. *J Clin Epidemiol*. 2012 Nov;65(11):1150–58.

Casarett DJ, Harrold J, Oldanie B, Prince-Paul M, Teno J. Advancing the science of hospice care: coalition of hospices organized to investigate comparative effectiveness. *Curr Opin Support Palliat Care*. 2012 Dec;6(4):459–64.

Chan A-W, Tetzlaff JM, Altman DG, et al. SPIRIT 2013 Statement: defining standard protocol items for clinical trials. *Ann Intern Med* 2013;158(3):200–07.

Chang SM, Carey TS, Kato EU, Guise JM, Sanders GD. Identifying research needs for improving health care. *Ann Intern Med*. 2012 Sep 18;157(6):439–45.

Charron S, Koechlin E. Divided representation of concurrent goals in the human frontal lobes. *Science*. 2010;328(5976):360–3.

Chernew ME, McKellar R, Aubry W, et al. Comparative effectiveness research and formulary placement: the case of diabetes. *Am J Manag Care*. 2013 Feb;19(2):93–96.

Chokshi DA, Avorn J, Kesselheim AS. Designing comparative effectiveness research on prescription drugs: lessons from the clinical trial literature. *Health Aff (Millwood)*. 2010;29(10):1842–48.

Chubak J, Rutter CM, Kamineni A, et al. Measurement in comparative effectiveness research. *Am J Prev Med*. 2013 May;44(5):513–19.

Clancy C, Collins FS. Patient-Centered Outcomes Research Institute: the intersection of science and health care. *Sci Transl Med*. 2010 Jun 23;2(37):37–18.

Clancy CM. Commentary: precision science and patient-centered care. *Acad Med*. 2011 Jun;86(6):667–70.

Conway PH, Clancy C. Charting a path from comparative effectiveness funding to improved patient-centered health care. *JAMA*. 2010 Mar 10;303(10):985–86.

Conway PH, Clancy C. Comparative-effectiveness research—implications of the Federal Coordinating Council's report. *N Engl J Med*. 2009 Jul 23;361(4):328–30.

De Moor MH, Boomsma DI, Stubbe JH, Willemsen G, de Geus EJ. Testing causality in the association between regular exercise and symptoms of anxiety and depression. *Arch Gen Psychiatry*. 2008 Aug;65(8):897–905.

Dentzer S; Editorial Team of Health Affairs. Communicating about comparative effectiveness research: a Health Affairs symposium on the issues. *Health Aff (Millwood)*. 2012 Oct;31(10):2183–87.

Des Jarlais DC, Lyles C, Crepaz N, and the TREND Group. Improving the reporting quality of nonrandomized evaluations of behavioral and public health interventions: the TREND statement. *Am J Public Health*. 2004;94(3):361–66.

Dreyer NA, Schneeweiss S, McNeil BJ, Berger ML, Walker AM, Ollendorf DA, Gliklich RE; GRACE Initiative. GRACE principles: recognizing high-quality observational studies of comparative effectiveness. *Am J Manag Care*. 2010 Jun;16(6):467–71.

Dubois RW, Graff JS. Setting priorities for comparative effectiveness research: from assessing public health benefits to being open with the public. *Health Aff (Millwood)*. 2011;30(12):2235–42.

Elwyn G, Frosch D, Thomson R, et al. Shared decision making: a model for clinical practice. *J Gen Intern Med*. 2012;27(10):1361–7.

Etheredge LM. Creating a high-performance system for comparative effectiveness research. *Health Aff (Millwood).* 2010;29(10):1761–67.

Eysenbach G; CONSORT-EHEALTH Group. CONSORT-EHEALTH: improving and standardizing evaluation reports of Web-based and mobile health interventions. *J Med Internet Res.* 2011 Dec 31;13(4):e126.

Farrington CP. Control without separate controls: evaluation of vaccine safety using case-only methods. *Vaccine.* 2004;22(15–16):2064–70.

Fendrick AM, Smith DG, Chernew ME. Applying value-based insurance design to low-value health services. *Health Aff (Millwood).* 2010 Nov;29(11):2017–21.

Fleurence RL, Naci H, Jansen JP. The critical role of observational evidence in comparative effectiveness research. *Health Aff (Millwood).* 2010;29(10):1826–33.

Forum, EDM. Building the electronic clinical data infrastructure to improve patient outcomes: CER project profiles. (2012). Issue Briefs and Reports. Paper 7. http://repository.academyhealth.org/edm_briefs/7.

Gagnier JJ, Boon H, Rochon P, Moher D, Barnes J, Bombardier C. Reporting randomized, controlled trials of herbal interventions: an elaborated CONSORT statement. *Ann Intern Med* 2006;144(5):364–67.

Ginsburg GS, Kuderer NM. Comparative effectiveness research, genomics-enabled personalized medicine, and rapid learning health care: a common bond. *J Clin Oncol.* 2012 Dec 1;30(34):4233–42.

Greenfield S, Kaplan SH. Building useful evidence: changing the clinical research paradigm to account for comparative effectiveness research. *J Comp Eff Res.* 2012;1(3):263–70.

Guyatt G, Oxman AD, Akl EA, et al. GRADE guidelines: 1. Introduction-GRADE evidence profiles and summary of findings tables. *J Clin Epidemiol.* 2011 Apr;64(4):383–94.

Guyatt GH, Oxman AD, Kunz R, et al. GRADE guidelines: 2. Framing the question and deciding on important outcomes. *J Clin Epidemiol.* 2011 Apr;64(4):395–400.

Guyatt GH, Oxman AD, Vist G, et al. GRADE guidelines: 4. Rating the quality of evidence—study limitations (risk of bias). *J Clin Epidemiol.* 2011 Apr;64(4):407–15.

Guyatt GH, Oxman AD, Montori V, et al. GRADE guidelines: 5. Rating the quality of evidence—publication bias. *J Clin Epidemiol.* 2011 Dec;64(12):1277–82.

Guyatt GH, Oxman AD, Kunz R, et al. GRADE guidelines 6. Rating the quality of evidence—imprecision. *J Clin Epidemiol.* 2011 Dec;64(12):1283–93.

Guyatt GH, Oxman AD, Kunz R, et al.; GRADE Working Group. GRADE guidelines: 7. Rating the quality of evidence—inconsistency. *J Clin Epidemiol.* 2011 Dec;64(12):1294–302.

Guyatt GH, Oxman AD, Kunz R, et al.; GRADE Working Group. GRADE guidelines: 8. Rating the quality of evidence—indirectness. *J Clin Epidemiol.* 2011 Dec;64(12):1303–10.

Guyatt GH, Oxman AD, Sultan S, et al.; GRADE Working Group. GRADE guidelines: 9. Rating up the quality of evidence. *J Clin Epidemiol.* 2011 Dec;64(12):1311–16.

Guyatt G, Oxman AD, Sultan S, et al. GRADE guidelines: 11. Making an overall rating of confidence in effect estimates for a single outcome and for all outcomes. *J Clin Epidemiol.* 2013 Feb;66(2):151–57.

Guyatt GH, Oxman AD, Santesso N, et al. GRADE guidelines: 12. Preparing summary of findings tables-binary outcomes. *J Clin Epidemiol.* 2013 Feb;66(2):158–72.

Guyatt GH, Thorlund K, Oxman AD, et al. GRADE guidelines: 13. Preparing summary of findings tables and evidence profiles-continuous outcomes. *J Clin Epidemiol.* 2013 Feb;66(2):173–83.

Hartung DM, Guise JM, Fagnan LJ, Davis MM, Stange KC. Role of practice-based research networks in comparative effectiveness research. *J Comp Eff Res.* 2012 Jan;1(1):45–55.

Hastings-Tolsma M, Matthews EE, Nelson JM, Schmiege S. Comparative effectiveness research: nursing science and health care delivery. *West J Nurs Res.* 2013 Jan 29. [Epub ahead of print]

Haynes AB, Weiser TG, Berry WR, et al.; Safe Surgery Saves Lives Study Group. A surgical safety checklist to reduce morbidity and mortality in a global population. *N Engl J Med.* 2009 Jan 29;360(5):491–9.

Herbst AL, Ulfelder H, Poskanzer DC. Adenocarcinoma of the vagina—association of maternal stilbestrol therapy with tumor appearance in young women. *N Engl J Med.* 1971; 284(15):878–881.

Hébert PC, Wells G, Blajchman MA, et al. A multicenter, randomized, controlled clinical trial of transfusion requirements in critical care. Transfusion Requirements in Critical Care Investigators, Canadian Critical Care Trials Group. *N Engl J Med.* 1999 Feb 11;340(6):409–17.

Hershman DL, Wright JD. Comparative effectiveness research in oncology methodology: observational data. *J Clin Oncol.* 2012 Dec 1;30(34):4215–22.

Hlatky MA, Winkelmayer WC, Setoguchi S. Epidemiologic and statistical methods for comparative effectiveness research. *Heart Fail Clin.* 2013 Jan;9(1):29–36.

Hoffman A, Montgomery R, Aubry W, Tunis SR. How best to engage patients, doctors, and other stakeholders in designing comparative effectiveness studies. *Health Aff (Millwood).* 2010;29(10):1834–41.

Hopewell S, Clarke M, Moher D, et al. and the CONSORT Group. CONSORT for reporting randomized controlled trials in journal and conference abstracts: explanation and elaboration. *PLoS Med* 2008;5(1):e20, doi:10.1371/journal.

Horn SD, Gassaway J. Practice-based evidence study design for comparative effectiveness research. *Med Care.* 2007 Oct;45(10 Supl 2):S50–7.

Huang SS, Septimus E, Kleinman K, et al.; CDC Prevention Epicenters Program; AHRQ DECIDE Network and Healthcare-Associated Infections Program. Targeted versus universal decolonization to prevent ICU infection. *N Engl J Med.* 2013 Jun 13;368(24):2255–65.

Husereau D, Drummond M, Petrou S, et al. Consolidated Health Economic Evaluation Reporting Standards (CHEERS) statement. *Eur J Health Econ.* 2013 Jun;14(3):367–72.

Institute of Medicine. *Health Literacy: A Prescription to End Confusion.* Washington, DC, National Academies Press, 2004.

Institute of Medicine. *Initial National Priorities for Comparative Effectiveness Research.* Washington, DC, National Academies Press, 2009.

Institute of Medicine. *Finding What Works in Health Care: Standards for Systematic Reviews.* Washington, DC, National Academies Press, 2011.

Ioannidis JP, Evans SJ, Gotzsche PC, et al. Better reporting of harms in randomized trials: an extension of the CONSORT statement. *Ann Intern Med* 2004;141(10):781–88.

Johnson ES, Bartman BA, Briesacher BA, et al. The incident user design in comparative effectiveness research. *Pharmacoepidemiol Drug Saf.* 2013 Jan;22(1):1–6.

Karnon J, Stahl J, Brennan A, Caro JJ, Mar J, Möller J; ISPOR-SMDM Modeling Good Research Practices Task Force. Modeling using discrete event simulation: a report of the ISPOR-SMDM Modeling Good Research Practices Task Force—4. *Value Health.* 2012 Sep–Oct;15(6):821–27.

Kelman CD. Phaco-emulsification and aspiration of senil cataracts: a comparative study with intra-capsular extraction. *Can J Ophthalmol.* 1973 Jan;8(1):24–32.

Kenney JT Jr. Managing the evolving complexity of pharmacologic treatment: comparative effectiveness research, pharmacoeconomic data analyses, and other decision support tools. *Am J Manag Care.* 2012 Nov;18(10 Suppl):S234–39.

Keren R, Luan X, Localio R, et al.; Pediatric Research in Inpatient Settings (PRIS) Network. Prioritization of comparative effectiveness research topics in hospital pediatrics. *Arch Pediatr Adolesc Med.* 2012 Dec;166(12):1155–64.

Lei H, Nahum-Shani I, Lynch K, Oslin D, Murphy SA. A "SMART" design for building individualized treatment sequences. *Annu Rev Clin Psychol.* 2012;8:21–48.

Li T, Vedula SS, Scherer R, Dickersin K. What comparative effectiveness research is needed? a framework for using guidelines and systematic reviews to identify evidence gaps and research priorities. *Ann Intern Med.* 2012 Mar 6;156(5):367–77.

Li YP, Fang LQ, Gao SQ, et al. Decision support system for the response to infectious disease emergencies based on WebGIS and mobile services in China. *PLoS One.* 2013;8(1):e54842.

Lofters AK, Gozdyra P, Lobb R. Using geographic methods to inform cancer screening interventions for South Asians in Ontario, Canada. *BMC Public Health.* 2013 Apr 26;13:395.

MacPherson H, Altman DG, Hammerschlag R, et al.; STRICTA Revision Group. Revised Standards for Reporting Interventions in Clinical Trials of Acupuncture (STRICTA): extending the CONSORT statement. *PLoS Med.* 2010 Jun 8;7(6):e1000261.

Maddux FW, Dickinson TA, Rilla D, et al. Institutional variability of intraoperative red blood cell utilization in coronary artery bypass graft surgery. *Am J Med Qual.* 2009 Sep-Oct;24(5):403–11.

McShane LM, Altman DG, Sauerbrei W, et al.; Statistics Subcommittee of the NCI-EORTC Working Group on Cancer Diagnostics. Reporting recommendations for tumor marker prognostic studies (REMARK). *J Natl Cancer Inst.* 2005 Aug 17;97(16):1180–84.

Methodology Committee of the Patient-Centered Outcomes Research Institute (PCORI). Methodological standards and patient-centeredness in comparative effectiveness research: the PCORI perspective. *JAMA.* 2012;307(15):1636–40.

Milton K, Clemes S, Bull F. Can a single question provide an accurate measure of physical activity? *Br J Sports Med.* 2013 Jan;47(1):44–8.

Miriovsky BJ, Shulman LN, Abernethy AP. Importance of health information technology, electronic health records, and continuously aggregating data to comparative effectiveness research and learning health care. *J Clin Oncol.* 2012 Dec 1;30(34):4243–48.

Moher D, Liberati A, Tetzlaff J, Altman DG, The PRISMA Group (2009). Preferred Reporting Items for Systematic Reviews and Meta-Analyses: the PRISMA Statement. *BMJ* 2009;339:b2535, doi: 10.1136/bmj.b2535.

Mullins CD, Abdulhalim AM, Lavallee DC. Continuous patient engagement in comparative effectiveness research. *JAMA.* 2012 Apr 18;307(15):1587–88.

Mushlin AI, Ghomrawi H. Health care reform and the need for comparative-effectiveness research. *N Engl J Med.* 2010 Jan 21;362(3):e6.

Mustafa RA, Santesso N, Brozek J, et al. The GRADE approach is reproducible in assessing the quality of evidence of quantitative evidence syntheses. *J Clin Epidemiol.* 2013 Jul;66(7):736–42.e5.

Ogrinc G, Mooney SE, Estrada C, et al. The SQUIRE (Standards for Quality Improvement Reporting Excellence) guidelines for quality improvement reporting: explanation and elaboration. *Qual Saf Health Care*. 2008 Oct;17(Suppl 1):i13–32.

Pace WD, Cifuentes M, Valuck RJ, Staton EW, Brandt EC, West DR. An electronic practice-based network for observational comparative effectiveness research. *Ann Intern Med*. 2009 Sep 1;151(5):338–40.

Piaggio G, Elbourne DR, Pocock SJ, Evans SJ, Altman DG; CONSORT Group. Reporting of noninferiority and equivalence randomized trials: extension of the CONSORT 2010 statement. *JAMA*. 2012 Dec 26;308(24):2594–604.

Pilkonis PA, Yu L, Colditz J, et al. Item banks for alcohol use from the Patient-Reported Outcomes Measurement Information System (PROMIS): use, consequences, and expectancies. *Drug Alcohol Depend*. 2013 Jun 1;130(1–3):167–77.

Pitman R, Fisman D, Zaric GS, et al.; ISPOR-SMDM Modeling Good Research Practices Task Force. Dynamic transmission modeling: a report of the ISPOR-SMDM Modeling Good Research Practices Task Force—5. *Value Health*. 2012 Sep–Oct;15(6):828–34.

Protti D, Johansen I. Widespread Adoption of Information Technology in Primary Care Physician Offices in Denmark: A Case Study, The Commonwealth Fund, March 2010.

Ramsey SD, Sullivan SD, Reed SD, et al. Oncology comparative effectiveness research: a multistakeholder perspective on principles for conduct and reporting. *Oncologist*. 2013 May 6. [Epub ahead of print]

Ranasinghe I, Turnbull F, Tonkin A, Clark RA, Coffee N, Brieger D. Comparative effectiveness of population interventions to improve access to reperfusion for ST-segment-elevation myocardial infarction in Australia. *Circ Cardiovasc Qual Outcomes*. 2012 Jul 1;5(4):429–36.

Reeve BB, Wyrwich KW, Wu AW, et al. ISOQOL recommends minimum standards for patient-reported outcome measures used in patient-centered outcomes and comparative effectiveness research. *Qual Life Res*. 2013 Jan 4. [Epub ahead of print]

Rogers MA, Small D, Buchan DA, et al. Home monitoring service improves mean arterial pressure in patients with essential hypertension. A randomized, controlled trial. *Ann Intern Med*. 2001 Jun 5;134(11):1024–32.

Saman DM, Johnson AO, Arevalo O, Odoi A. Geospatially illustrating regional-based oral health disparities in Kentucky. *Public Health Rep*. 2011;126(4):612–8.

Schulz KF, Altman DG, Moher D; CONSORT Group. CONSORT 2010 statement: updated guidelines for reporting parallel group randomised trials. *PLoS Med*. 2010 Mar 24;7(3):e1000251.

Segal JB, Kapoor W, Carey T, et al. Preliminary competencies for comparative effectiveness research. *Clin Transl Sci*. 2012 Dec;5(6):476–79.

Selby JV, Beal AC, Frank L. The Patient-Centered Outcomes Research Institute (PCORI) national priorities for research and initial research agenda. *JAMA*. 2012;307(15):1583–84.

Silveira MJ, Connor SR, Goold SD, McMahon LF, Feudtner C. Community supply of hospice: does wealth play a role? *J Pain Symptom Manage*. 2011 Jul;42(1):76–82.

Simonds NI, Khoury MJ, Schully SD, et al. Comparative effectiveness research in cancer genomics and precision medicine: current landscape and future prospects. *J Natl Cancer Inst*. 2013 May 9. [Epub ahead of print]

Simpson LA, Peterson L, Lannon CM, et al. Special challenges in comparative effectiveness research on children's and adolescents' health. *Health Aff (Millwood)*. 2010;29(10):1849–56.

Slichter SJ, Kaufman RM, Assmann SF, et al. Dose of prophylactic platelet transfusions and prevention of hemorrhage. *N Engl J Med*. 2010 Feb 18;362(7):600–13.

Snyder CF, Aaronson NK, Choucair AK, et al. Implementing patient-reported outcomes assessment in clinical practice: a review of the options and considerations. *Qual Life Res*. 2012 Oct;21(8):1305–14.

Stewart JE, Battersby SE, Lopez-De Fede A, et al. Diabetes and the socioeconomic and built environment: geovisualization of disease prevalence and potential contextual associations using ring maps. *Int J Health Geogr*. 2011 Mar 1;10:18.

Sullivan SD, Carlson JJ, Hansen RN. Comparative effectiveness research in the United States: a progress report. *J Med Econ*. 2013;16(2):295–97.

Teno JM, Gozalo PL, Bynum JP, et al. Change in end-of-life care for Medicare beneficiaries: site of death, place of care, and health care transitions in 2000, 2005, and 2009. *JAMA*. 2013 Feb 6;309(5):470–7.

Teutsch SM, Fielding JE. Applying comparative effectiveness research to public and population health initiatives. *Health Aff (Millwood)*. 2011 Feb;30(2):349–55.

Thorpe KE, Zwarenstein M, Oxman AD, et al. A pragmatic-explanatory continuum indicator summary (PRECIS): a tool to help trial designers. *CMAJ*. 2009 May 12;180(10):E47-57.

Thorpe KE, Zwarenstein M, Oxman AD, et al. A pragmatic-explanatory continuum indicator summary (PRECIS): a tool to help trial designers. *J Clin Epidemiol*. 2009 May;62(5):464–75.

Tinetti ME, Studenski SA. Comparative effectiveness research and patients with multiple chronic conditions. *N Engl J Med*. 2011 Jun 30;364(26):2478–81.

Tong A, Flemming K, McInnes E, Oliver S, Craig J. Enhancing transparency in reporting the synthesis of qualitative research: ENTREQ. *BMC Med Res Methodol*. 2012 Nov 27;12:181.

Tong A, Sainsbury P, Craig J. Consolidated criteria for reporting qualitative research (COREQ): a 32-item checklist for interviews and focus groups. *Int J Qual Health Care*. 2007 Dec;19(6):349–57.

Tunis SR, Stryer DB, Clancy CM. Practical clinical trials: increasing the value of clinical research for decision making in clinical and health policy. *JAMA*. 2003;290(12):1624–32.

Tunis SR, Turkelson C. Using health technology assessment to identify gaps in evidence and inform study design for comparative effectiveness research. *J Clin Oncol*. 2012 Dec 1;30(34):4256–61.

VanLare JM, Conway PH, Sox HC. Five next steps for a new national program for comparative-effectiveness research. *N Engl J Med*. 2010;362(11):970–73.

Van Spall HG, Toren A, Kiss A, Fowler RA. Eligibility criteria of randomized controlled trials published in high-impact general medical journals: a systematic sampling review. *JAMA*. 2007;297(11):1233–40.

von Elm E, Altman DG, Egger M, Pocock SJ, Gøtzsche PC, Vandenbroucke JP; STROBE Initiative. The Strengthening the Reporting of Observational Studies in Epidemiology (STROBE) statement: guidelines for reporting observational studies. *J Clin Epidemiol*. 2008 Apr;61(4):344–49.

Wangia V, Shireman TI. A review of geographic variation and Geographic Information Systems (GIS) applications in prescription drug use research. *Res Social Adm Pharm.* 2013 Jan 17. pii: S1551-7411(12)00359-2.

Weber SC, Seto T, Olson C, Kenkare P, Kurian AW, Das AK. Oncoshare: lessons learned from building an integrated multi-institutional database for comparative effectiveness research. *AMIA Annu Symp Proc.* 2012;2012:970-78.

Wennberg JE. *Tracking Medicine: A Researcher's Quest to Understand Health Care.* New York, Oxford University Press, 2010.

Wilson DS, Dapic V, Sultan DH, et al. Establishing the infrastructure to conduct comparative effectiveness research toward the elimination of disparities: a community-based participatory research framework. *Health Promot Pract.* 2013 Feb 21. [Epub ahead of print]

Witt CM. Clinical research on traditional drugs and food items—the potential of comparative effectiveness research for interdisciplinary research. *J Ethnopharmacol.* 2013 May 2;147(1):254-58.

Witt CM, Chesney M, Gliklich R, et al. Building a strategic framework for comparative effectiveness research in complementary and integrative medicine. *Evid Based Complement Alternat Med.* 2012:531096.

Wu AW, Snyder C, Clancy CM, Steinwachs DM. Adding the patient perspective to comparative effectiveness research. *Health Aff (Millwood).* 2010;29(10):1863-71.

Zwarenstein M, Treweek S, Gagnier JJ, et al. for the CONSORT and Pragmatic Trials in Healthcare (Practihc) group. Improving the reporting of pragmatic trials: an extension of the CONSORT statement. *BMJ* 2008; 337;a2390.

INDEX

absolute risk difference, 56
abstracts
   Biological Abstracts, 15
   of conferences, 174
   databases of, 112
   of journal articles, 14
   of reviews of effects, 14
   See also databases; search engines.
adaptive trials
   CONSORT (Consolidated Standards of Reporting Trials), 75
   eligibility criteria, 73
   fixed sample size, 74–75
   fixed-size randomized trials, 74–75
   interim analysis showing beneficial effect, 74
   interim analysis showing lack of effect, 74
   overview, 73
   randomization, 74
   sequential randomized controlled trials, 75
   SMART (sequential multiple assignment randomized trial), 75
   study populations, 74
   unexpected outcomes, 73–74
adherence, as comparator, 40–41
ADLs (basic activities of daily living), 46
administration, measurement instruments, 52
adverse effects, 25
age, in study participants, 126
Agency for Healthcare Research and Quality
   National Quality Measure Clearinghouse, 51
   Patients & Consumers, 180
aging, 108
Aging Integrated Database, 108
AGRICOLA, 15
AGRIS (International Information System for the Agricultural Sciences and Technology), 15
AHRQ Health IT, YouTube channel, 27
alcohol intake in study participants, 129
allergenics studies. *See* biologics.
American FactFinder, 107
AMSTAR (Assessment of Multiple Systematic Reviews), 175
Annals of Internal Medicine, 120
antitoxin studies. *See* biologics.

anxiety, measuring patient-reported outcomes, 49
Archimedes Model, 160
Area Health Resource File, 109
armed forces members, in cohort studies, 99–100
arms
   adding during implementation, 73
   definition, 63
   parallel, 63
ASA24 Automated Self-administered 24-hour Recall site, 36
asbestos exposure, patient registries, 132
aspirin, decision aid for, 179
Assessment of Multiple Systematic Reviews (AMSTAR), 175
asthma, measuring patient-reported outcomes, 51
Australian New Zealand Clinical Trials Registry, 169
Australian Society of Cardiac Surgeons, patient registry, 132

BADLs (basic activities of daily living), 46
Bandolier site, 58
Barthel Index, 46
BASE (Bielefeld Academic Search Engine), 16, 17
basic activities of daily living (ADLs), 46
basic activities of daily living (BADLs), 46
Bayesian inference, evaluating outcomes, 58–59
Behavioral Risk Factor Surveillance System, 131
behavioral sciences, bibliographic database, 15
Belmont Report, 167–169
between-person comparisons, 65
bias
   children in samples, 24
   in clinical drug trials, 24
   individuals with multiple diseases, 24
   in large databases, 161
   older adults in samples, 24
   selection, 161
   women in samples, 24
bibliographic databases
   abstracts of journal articles, 14
   abstracts of reviews of effects, 14

bibliographic databases (*Cont.*)
  AGRICOLA, 15
  AGRIS (International Information System for the Agricultural Sciences and Technology), 15
  behavioral sciences, 15
  Biological Abstracts, 15
  biomedical publications, 16
  biomedical research, 14
  CINAHL (Cumulative Index to Nursing and Allied Health Literature), 15
  Cochrane Library, 14
  Collection of Computer Science Bibliographies, 15
  digital library resources, 15
  drug therapies, 14
  economic aspects of health care, 15
  educational literature, 15
  Embase, 14
  ERIC (Education Resources Information Center), 15, 17
  Food and Agriculture Organization of the United Nations, 15
  health technology assessment, 14
  injury research, 16
  MEDLINE, 14
  mental health, 15
  MeSH (Medical Subject Headings), 14
  methodology register, 14
  National Health System economic evaluation, 14
  nursing and allied professions, 15
  nutrition and diet, 15
  patient-reported outcomes, 50
  peer reviewed literature, 15
  pharmacologic studies, 14
  Physiotherapy Evidence Database, 15
  psychology, 15, 112
  PsycINFO, 15, 112
  RefPRO, 50
  register of controlled trials, 14
  RePEc (Research Papers in Economics), 15
  SafetyLit, 16
  SciELO (Scientific Electronic Library Online), 16
  scientific literature, 15
  Scopus, 15
  social aspects of health and disease, 16
  Social Science Research Network, 16
  systematic reviews, 14
  Web of Science, 15
  WorldCat, 15
Bielefeld Academic Search Engine (BASE), 16, 17
Bioinformatic Harvester, 18
Biological Abstracts database, 15
biologics
  ClinicalTrials.gov, 30
  as comparators, 28–31
  drugs *vs.*, 28–29
  gene therapy, 30
  Human Microbiome Project, 30
  human microbiota, 30
  ICTRP (International Clinical Trials Registry), 30
  International Human Microbiome Consortium, 30
  Metagenomics of the Human Intestinal Tract, 30
  microbiome sites, 30
  microorganisms, 30
  plasmid therapies, 31
  regulatory agency, 29
  stem cell therapy, 30
  storage and administration, 29
  vaccines, 29–30
  virus therapies, 31
biomedical literature, search engine, 18
biomedical original research articles, search engine, 16
biomedical publications database, 16
biomedical research database, 14
birth cohorts, 99
blinding, 64–65
blocking, trial design, 69–70, 71
block size, determining, 70–71
blood and blood product studies. *See* biologics.
blood disorders, 185
blood transfusions
  individual differences, 29
  red blood cells, 185
  risks and benefits, 185
  TRICC (Transfusion Requirements in Critical Care) trial, 185
  triggers, 185
blood transfusion thresholds, 185
books and publications
  Annals of Internal Medicine, 120
  "Comparative Efficacy of Seven Psychotherapeutic Interventions for Patients with Depression…," 39
  Dartmouth Atlas of Health Care, 22, 135, 139
  Dartmouth Atlas of Health Care online, 138
  "Evaluating Test Strategies for Colorectal Cancer Screening…," 120
  The Guide to Clinical Preventive Services, 156
  Health Affairs, 157
  "Instrumental Variable Methods in Comparative Safety and Effectiveness Research," 88
  Medical Care, 157

Milbank Quarterly, 157
New England Journal of Medicine, 185
"Shared Decision Making: A Model for Clinical Practice," 6
"Toward Precision Medicine: Building a Knowledge Network for Biomedical Research and a New Taxonomy of Disease," 122
WHO world report on disability, 53
See also specific books and publications.
British Doctors Study, 99
built environment
   effects on health, 137–138
   exercise and mobility, 37–38
burden, measurement instruments, 52

Canadian Agency for Drugs and Technologies in Health Care, 9
Canadian Joint Replacement Registry, patient registry, 132
Canadian Task Force on Preventive Health Care, 156
cancer
   breast, 143–144
   colorectal, 120
   geographic distribution, 139
   precision medicine, 123
   screening, 120
   time issues, 143–144
cardiac care
   Australian Society of Cardiac Surgeons, 132
   European Cardiac Surgical Registry, 132
   Framingham Heart Study, 90
   Interactive Atlas of Heart Disease and Stroke, 136
   Society of Thoracic Surgeons National Database, 132
care transition
   search engine, 17
   type 1 diabetes, 10, 16, 17
case-control studies, checklists, 174
case-crossover design
   description, 91–93
   institutionalized settings, 153
cataract surgery, 186
CDC (Center for Disease Control and Prevention)
   Behavioral Risk Factor Surveillance System, 131
   Gateway to Health Communication & Social Marketing Practice, 180
   health literacy, 6
   Injury Statistics Query and Reporting System, 97
   Inpatient Surgery site, 32

NHANES (National Health and Nutrition Examination Survey), 35
   presenting information, 4
   Public-Use Data files and Documentation, 102
   Smoking & Tobacco Use Surveys, 130
   Surveys and Data Collection Systems, 108
   Wonder, 109
cellular products studies. *See* biologics.
census data, databases of, 109
Center for Longitudinal Studies, 99
Center for Medical Technology Policy, 164
Centers for Medicare and Medicade Services, 102
CenterWatch.com, 24
CENTRAL (Cochrane Central Register of Controlled Trials), 24, 112
CERTs (Centers for Education and Research on Therapeutics), 178
CESSDA (Council of European Social Science Data Archives), 110
checklists
   case-control studies, 174
   cohort studies, 174
   conference abstracts, 174
   CONSORT, 172–173
   cross-sectional studies, 174
   definition, 44
   depression measurements, 45
   PHQ9 (Patient Health Questionnaire depression module 9), 45
   reporting and publishing randomized trials, 172–173
   SPIRIT, 173–174
   STROBE, 174
   surgical procedures, 31–32
   of symptoms, 45
   trial protocols, 173–174
   World Health Organization Surgical Safety Checklist, 31
   See also measurement instruments; questionnaires.
CHEERS (Consolidated Health Economic Evaluation Reporting Standards), 174
children
   international research, 110–111
   nutrition, 110
   sample biases, 24
   Women, Infants, and Children program, 110
children, measurement instruments
   chronic illnesses, 46
   developmental scales, 46
   Pediatric Quality of Life Inventory, 47–48
cholera epidemic, London, 88, 135
Choosing Wisely program, 19–20
Chronic Conditions Data Warehouse, 103

chronic illness
  in children, measurement instruments, 46
  database of, 103
  dietary research, 35–36
CINAHL (Cumulative Index to Nursing and Allied Health Literature), 15, 112
CiteSeer search engine, 16
clinical drug trials
  adverse effects, 25
  CenterWatch.com, 24
  CENTRAL (Cochrane Central Register for Controlled Trials), 24
  ClinicalTrials.gov, 24
  common shortcomings, 24
  designing, 83
  International Clinical Trials Registry Platform, 24
  phases, 23–24
  registering, 24
  sample biases, 24
  side effects, 25
  Web site, 23–24
  See also outcomes; studies of specific therapies.
Clinical Queries, 154
clinical trails registry database, 53
Clinical Trails Registry Platform, 53
ClinicalTrials.gov, 24, 30, 169
cluster comparisons, 65–66
cluster randomized trials
  example, 76
  overview, 76
  REDUCE MRSA trial, 76
  sequential enrollment, 77
  stepped wedge design, 76–78
Cochrane, Archibald, 112
Cochrane Central Register of Controlled Trials (CENTRAL), 24, 112
Cochrane Collaboration, 9, 112
Cochrane Handbook for Systematic Reviews of Interventions online, 112
Cochrane Library database, 14, 17
Cochrane Summaries site, 32
cognition, measuring patient-reported outcomes, 51
cognitive behavioral therapy, 38
cohort studies
  birth cohorts, 99
  British Doctors Study, 99
  Center for Longitudinal Studies, 99
  checklists, 174
  common experiences, patient registry, 133
  comprehensive cohort trial design, 86–87
  decision modeling, 119
  definition, 97–98
  designing, 97–100
  institutionalized settings, 152–153
  members of the armed forces, 99–100
  Millennium Cohort Study, 99
  National Children's Study, 99
  natural cohorts, 99–100
  Nurse's Health Study, 99
  overview, 97–98
  pregnant women, 99
  retrospective *vs.* prospective, 98
  types of, 99
cold/heat therapy, as comparator, 41
Collection of Computer Science Bibliographies, 15
colorectal cancer screening, 120
Community Clinical Trial System, 170
comparability, measurement instruments, 52
comparative effectiveness research
  areas of need, 7
  definition, 3
  distinguishing features, 4
  funding, effects on focus, 7–8
  funding, effects on priorities, 13–14
  future of, 183–186
  general steps in, 166–167
  head-to-head comparisons, 3
  objective of, 6
  purpose of, 3
  review summaries, 178
  roots of, 8–9
  See also guidelines for comparative effectiveness research.
Comparative Effectiveness Review Summary Guides, 178
"Comparative Efficacy of Seven Psychotherapeutic Interventions for Patients with Depression...," 39
comparators
  adherence, 40–41
  biologics, 28–31
  delivery systems, 39–40
  diet and food, 34–36
  education, 42
  exercise and mobility, 37–38
  extraneous factors *vs.*, 90–91
  heat/cold therapy, 41
  information technologies, 27–28
  location as, 140
  medical devices, 25–27
  medications, 23–25
  nonhuman, 41
  pets, 41
  placebos, 21–22
  psychotherapeutic approaches, 38–39
  screening tests, 32–33

shoes, 41
social support, 38–39
surgical procedures, 31–32
   in twins, 105
   usual care, 22–23
complex modeling, large databases, 160–161
comprehensive cohort trial design, 86–87
Comprehensive Epidemiologic Data Resource site, 110
concealed randomization, 65
conferences
   abstracts, checklist, 174
   proceedings, databases of, 112
confidence intervals, evaluating outcomes, 57–58
confounding factors, 66, 161–162
consent forms, 169
consequences. *See* outcomes.
Consolidated Health Economic Evaluation Reporting Standards (CHEERS), 174
CONSORT (Consolidated Standards of Reporting Trials), 75, 172–173
construct validity, 52
content validity, 52
contrast approach to selecting a study design, 162
contrasting groups, evaluating outcomes, 55
controls, in trials, 63
COREQ (Consolidated Criteria for Reporting Qualitative Research), 175
cost of health care, 32, 97, 108
Council for International Organizations of Medical Sciences, 169
Council of European Social Science Data Archives (CESSDA), 110
County Health Rankings, 136
criterion validity, 52
Critical Path Institute, 50–51
crossover effects, N-of-1 trials, 81
crossover trials
   issues, 79–80
   overview, 78
   within-person design, 78
cross-sectional studies, checklists, 174
Cumulative Index to Nursing and Allied Health Literature (CINAHL), 15, 112
cumulative meta-analysis, 116–117
Cystic Fibrosis Foundation, 132

daily activities, measurement instruments
   ADLs (basic activities of daily living), 46
   BADLs (basic activities of daily living), 46
   IADLs (instrumental activities of daily living), 46
   overview, 46–49
Danish Twin Registry, 132

Dartmouth Atlas of Health Care, 22, 135, 139
Dartmouth Atlas of Health Care online, 138
Data Archive of the Robert Wood Johnson Foundation, 158
databases
   abstracts, 112
   Aging Integrated Database, 108
   Area Health Resource File, 109
   CDC Public-Use Data files and Documentation, 102
   CDC Wonder, 109
   census data, 109
   Centers for Medicare and Medicade Services, 102
   CENTRAL (Cochrane Central Register of Controlled Trials), 112
   CESSDA (Council of European Social Science Data Archives), 110
   Chronic Conditions Data Warehouse, 103
   CINAHL (Cumulative Index to Nursing and Allied Health Literature), 112
   clinical trails registry, 53
   Clinical Trails Registry Platform, 53
   Cochrane Library, 17
   Comprehensive Epidemiologic Data Resource site, 110
   conference proceedings, 112
   data extraction tools, 111
   DataFerrett, 111
   DHHS Data Resources, 157
   disease burden, 110
   dissertations, 112
   Embase, 112
   Emergency Response Safety and Health Database, 110
   environmental factors, 110
   EU-ADR project, 98
   of food content, 36
   Food Distribution Programs, 110
   Framingham Heart Study, 103
   generated from registries, 103
   Global Health Data Exchange, 111
   Global Health Observatory, 110–111
   grey literature, 112
   HCUP (Healthcare Cost and Utilization Project), 32, 97, 108
   Health and Retirement Study, 103
   health care providers, 102
   HealthData.gov, 108
   Health for All Database, 110
   Health Improvement Network, 98
   Health Indicators Warehouse, 109
   Health Professional Shortage Areas, 109
   Health Resources and Service Administration, 109

Index **201**

databases (*Cont.*)
 health systems, 110
 hospital data, 108
 hospital inpatient information, 108
 immunizations, 110
 infectious diseases, 110
 injuries, 110
 Integrated Public Use Microdata Series, 109
 Integrated Public Use Microdata Series International, 109
 international health research, 110–111
 International Household Survey Network, 111
 International Human Development Indicators, 111
 Inter-University Consortium for Political and Social Research, 109
 Kaiser Permanente clinical research, 102
 Kids' Inpatient Database, 108
 longitudinal, 102–103, 159
 longitudinal studies, 98
 MEDLINE (Medical Literature Analysis and Retrieval System online), 111–112
 Millennium Development Goals Indicators, 111
 mortality, 110
 National Cancer Institute, 103
 National Center for Health Statistics Data Linkage Activities, 102
 National Institute for Occupational Safety and Health, 110
 national insurance records, 102
 National Quality Measures Clearinghouse, 109
 National Sample Survey of Registered Nurses, 109
 National Technical Information Services, 112
 Nationwide Emergency Department Sample, 108
 Nationwide Inpatient Sample, 108
 Netherland Information Network of General Practice, 98
 noninfectious diseases, 110
 nutrition data, 110
 Open Grey, 112
 original research studies, 111–112
 Partners in Information Access for the Public Health Workforce, 108
 PICO search, 11
 population data, 110
 predicting outcomes, 184
 Primary Care Service Areas, 109
 PROQOLID (Patient-Reported Outcome and Quality of Life Instruments Database), 50
 public health data, 102, 108–111
 Public-Use Data files and Documentation, 102
 ResDAC (Research Data Assistance Center), 103
 School Meals, 110
 SEER (Surveillance, Epidemiology, and End Results) program, 98, 103
 Society of Thoracic Surgeons National Database, 132
 SodaPop (PennState Online Data Archive for Population Studies), 109
 for specific diseases, 110
 State Ambulatory Surgery Databases, 108
 Supplemental Nutrition Assistance Program, 110
 theses, 112
 TRIP, 11, 17
 University HealthSystem Consortium, 102
 USDA nutrition programs, 110
 violence, 110
 WHO Clinical Trails Registry Platform, 53
 WHO Global Health Observatory, 110–111
 WHO Health for All Database, 110
 WISQARS (Web-Based Injury Statistics Query and Reporting System), 109
 Women, Infants, and Children program, 110
 Wonder, 109
 World Bank, 110
 See also bibliographic databases; patient registries; search engines; *specific databases*.
databases, large
 bias, 161
 complex modeling, 160–161
 confounding, 161–162
 data capabilities, 159
 information bias, 161
 instrumental variables, 161–162
 level of detail, 160
 longitudinal structure, 159
 multivariable adjustment, 161
 opportunity for discovery, 160–161
 overview, 158–159
 propensity analyses, 161
 selection bias, 161
 types of services, 159–160
data extraction tools, 111
DataFerrett, 111
data management in clinical research, 175–176
Data Resources of the DHHS, 157
DECIDE (Developing and Evaluating Communication Strategies to Support Informed Decisions and Practices Based on Evidence), 178

decision aids
   Agency for Healthcare Research and Quality, 180
   aspirin, 179
   Mayo Clinic, 179
   Ottawa Hospital Research Institute, 180
   statins, 179
decision making
   computational approach, 184
   online resources, 6
   "Shared Decision Making: A Model for Clinical Practice," 6
decision modeling
   cohorts of people over time, 119
   decision trees, 118–119
   discrete event simulation, 119
   events over time, 119
   future risk, 119–120
   HealthBound, 120
   Health Forecasting, 119–120
   health policy studies, 158
   Markov models, 119
   microsumulation, 119–120
   MISCAN (MIcrosimulation for Screening Analysis), 119
   Monte Carlo simulation, 119
   overview, 118
   POHEM (Population Health Model), 119–120
   ReThink Health, 120
decision trees, 118–119, 158
Declaration of Helsinki, 169
delayed start trials, 84
delivery systems, as comparator, 39–40
demographic information, gathering, 107
dental care, 186
Department of Energy search engine, 18
Department of Health and Human Services (DHHS). See DHHS (Department of Health and Human Services).
dependent variables. See outcomes.
depression
   measurement checklists, 45
   measuring patient-reported outcomes, 49, 51
   treating, 39
designing studies. See study design; trial design.
Design trumps analysis, 62
Developing and Evaluating Communication Strategies to Support Informed Decisions and Practices Based on Evidence (DECIDE), 178
Developing Evidence to Inform Decisions about Effectiveness Network, 178–179
developmental scales for children, 46
DHHS (Department of Health and Human Services)
   Data Resources, 157, 158
   Health Insurance Marketplace, 40
   Health Resources and Services Administration, 109
   Patient Protection and Affordable Care Act, 40
diabetes. See type 1 diabetes.
diaries, as measurement instruments, 45
diet and food
   as comparators, 34–36
   databases of food content, 36
   food frequency questionnaires, 35
   food records, 34
   24-hour dietary recall, 34
   NHANES (National Health and Nutrition Examination Survey), 35
   population differences, 35
   recording dietary intake, 34–35
   See also nutrition.
dietary research
   chronic disease studies, 35–36
   in developing countries, 35
   Iowa State University, 36
   NAT (Nutrition Analysis Tool), 36
   obstetrics and pediatrics, 35
   pregnancy, 35
   software for dietary intake, 36
   University of Illinois, 36
   University of Minnesota, 36
Diet History Questionnaire, 35–36
difference, medical definition, 56
differences between two measures, 55
digital library resources, database, 15
Directory of Open Access Journals, 16
disability
   measurement instruments, 53
   world report on, 53
disaster assistance, 110
discrete event simulation, 119, 158
disease
   databases of, 110
   incidence, rates of, 53
   prevention, patient registry, 132
disease burden
   databases of, 110
   measuring, 52–53
dissertations, databases of, 112
doctors. See physicians.
dose response trials, 83–84
drugs
   biologics vs., 28–29
   measuring patient-reported outcomes, 50
   phased clinical trials. See clinical drug trials.
   therapies, database of, 14
   use, geographic variations, 137
   See also medications.

drugs, searching by
    active ingredients, 24
    contraindications, 24
    name, 24
    recommended uses, 24
dynamic modeling, 158

EarthRisk Technologies, 141
economic aspects of health care, database, 15
educating patients and populations, 179–181
education, as comparator, 42
educational literature database, 15
Education Resources Information Center (ERIC), 15, 17
effectiveness *vs.* efficacy, 20–21
effects. *See* outcomes.
eHealth, 27–28
Electronic Patient Reported Outcome (ePRO) Consortium, 51
Embase, 14, 16, 112
emergency assistance, 110
emergency preparedness, effects on health, 138
Emergency Response Safety and Health Database, 110
emergency services, study design, 153–154
endpoints. *See* outcomes.
ENTREQ (Enhancing Transparency in Reporting the Synthesis of Qualitative Research), 174–175
environmental factors, databases of, 110
environmental health, patient registry, 132
epidemiology
    cholera epidemic, London, 88, 135
    MOOSE (Meta-Analysis of Observational Studies in Epidemiology), 172
    SEER (Surveillance, Epidemiology, and End Results) program, 98, 103
    STROBE (Strengthening the Reporting of Observational Studies in Epidemiology), 174
ePRO (Electronic Patient Reported Outcome) Consortium, 51
equalizing
    identical twins, 67
    trial groups, 69–70
equivalence trials, 84–85
ERIC (Education Resources Information Center), 15, 17
estimates of effect, 55
estrogen replacement, case study, 1
ethical principles for treatment of human subjects, 167–169
ethnicity in study participants, 127–129
EU-ADR project, 98
EudraCT, 170

European Cardiac Surgical Registry, 132
European Medicines Agency, 23
European portal of the WHO, 158
Europe PubMed Central, 17
EUROQol, 46
"Evaluating Test Strategies for Colorectal Cancer Screening...," 120
evidence
    assigning levels to, 171
    Physiotherapy Evidence Database, 15
    practice-based evidence studies, 100
evidence, incorporating into practice
    educating patients and populations, 179–181
    exploration stage, 176–177
    fill implementation stage, 177
    initial implementation stage, 177
    installation stage, 177
    methods for diffusion, 177–179
    National Implementation Research Network, 176–177
    stages of implementation, 176–177
evidence-based medicine, 9
Evidence-based Practice Centers, 178
exercise and mobility
    in built environments, 37–38
    as comparators, 37–38
    measurement instruments, 46
    physical activity in study participants, 130–131
    questionnaires, 37
experimentation *vs.* observation, 89–91
explanatory trials, 72
exploration stage, 176–177
eye health and vision
    cataract surgery, 186
    measurement instruments, 47

factorial trials, 82
factors, commonly studied. *See* comparators.
family medical history questionnaire, 131–132
fatigue, measuring patient-reported outcomes, 49
FDA (Food and Drug Administration)
    biologics regulation, 29
    For Consumers, 180
    medical device safety, 25
    National Medical Device Registry, 132
    organ transplants, 29
    responsibilities, 23
    Unique Device Identification System, 132
fill implementation stage, 177
filtering search engine results, 18
fixed-size randomized trials, 74–75
food. *See* diet and food; nutrition.

Food and Agriculture Organization of the
    United Nations, 15
Food Distribution Programs, 110
food frequency questionnaires, 35
food records, 34
For Consumers, 180
forest plots, 116–117
Framingham Heart Study, 103
Functional Assessment of Chronic Illness
    Therapy, 47
functioning, measurement instruments, 46–49
funding, effects on research
    focus of questions, 7–8
    priorities, 13–14

gap method to selecting a study design, 163–164
gene products studies. *See* biologics.
gene therapy, 30
genetic studies, search engine, 18
genetic traits, 122
Genome-wide Association Studies, 51
genotypes, 122
GIS (Geographic Information Systems), 137–139
global health, measuring patient-reported
    outcomes, 49
Global Health Data Exchange, 111
Global Health Observational Map Gallery, 139
Global Health Observatory, 110–111
Global Observatory, 158
good health, definition of, 43
Google Scholar search engine, 16
GRACE Principles, 174
GRADE (Grading of Recommendations
    Assessment, Development, and
    Evaluation), 170–171
GRADE Working Group, 171
grey literature, databases of, 112
guidelines for comparative effectiveness research
    AMSTAR (Assessment of Multiple
        Systematic Reviews), 175
    CHEERS (Consolidated Health Economic
        Evaluation Reporting Standards), 174
    CONSORT (Consolidated Standards of
        Reporting Trials), 172–173
    COREQ (Consolidated Criteria for
        Reporting Qualitative Research), 175
    ENTREQ (Enhancing Transparency in
        Reporting the Synthesis of Qualitative
        Research), 174–175
    GRADE (Grading of Recommendations
        Assessment, Development, and
        Evaluation), 170–171
    MOOSE (Meta-Analysis of Observational
        Studies in Epidemiology), 172
    overview, 170
    PRISMA (Preferred Reporting Items for
        Systematic Reviews and Meta-Analyses),
        171–172
    QUADAS (Quality Assessment of Diagnostic
        Accuracy Studies), 175
    SPIRIT (Standard Protocol Items:
        Recommendations for Interventional
        Trials), 173–174
    SQUIRE (Standards for Quality
        Improvement Reporting Excellence), 175
    STARD (Standards for the Reporting of
        Diagnostic Accuracy Studies), 175
    STROBE (Strengthening the Reporting of
        Observational Studies in Epidemiology),
        174
    TREND (Transparent Reporting of
        Evaluations Nonrandomized Designs),
        174
The Guide to Clinical Preventive Services, 156

HCUP (Healthcare Cost and Utilization
    Project), 32, 97, 108
head-to-head comparisons, 3
Health Affairs, 157
Health and Activities Limitations Index, 47
Health and Medical Care Archive, 158
Health and Retirement Study, 101, 103
HealthBound, 120
Health Canada, 23
health care providers
    databases of, 102
    workforce, effects on health, 138
    See also nurses; physicians.
Health Care Systems Research Collaboratory, 75
HealthData.gov, 108
healthfinder.gov, 180
Health for All Database, 110
Health Forecasting, 119–120
Health Improvement Network, 98
Health Indicators Warehouse, 109
Health Insurance Marketplace, 40
HealthIT, 28
HealthIT AHRQ site, 27
health literacy, 6
HealthMap, 139
HealthMap Vaccine Finder, 139
health policies, study design, 157–158
Health Professional Shortage Areas, 109
health-related data surveys, 108–111
health-related maps, 136
health-related quality of life, 46–49
health-relevant lifestyle factors in study
    participants, 128–129
Health Resources and Services Administration,
    29, 109

health services access, effects on health, 137
health systems, databases of, 110
health technology assessment database, 14
Health Utilities Index, 46–47
healthy lifespan, 52–53
heart health. *See* cardiac care.
heat/cold therapy, as comparator, 41
Henry J. Kaiser Family Foundation, 136
heterogeneity, meta-analysis, 117
home health services, study design, 155
hospitals
    databases of, 108
    designing studies for, 152–153
    in-hospital mortality, 147
    inpatient information, 108
    length of stay, 146–147
    statistics, 97
24-hour dietary recall, 34
HubMed search engine, 17
Human Microbiome Project, 30
human microbiota, as therapy, 30
human subjects. *See* study participants.
hydroxyurea, case study, 1
hysterectomy, case study, 1

IADLs (instrumental activities of daily living), 46
IBM Watson, 160, 184
ICTRP (International Clinical Trials Registry Platform), 24, 30, 170
immunizations, databases of, 110
    See also vaccines.
independent variables. *See* comparators.
infant mortality, by country, 53
infants
    nutrition, 110
    Women, Infants, and Children program, 110
infection process, time issues, 143
infectious diseases
    databases of, 110
    modeling, 138
influence assessment, meta-analysis, 117
information bias in large databases, 161
information science, search engine, 16
information technologies, as comparator, 27–28
Informed Medical Decisions Foundation, 6
inherited traits *vs.* genetic, 122
initial implementation stage, 177
Initial National Priorities for Comparative Effectiveness Research, 151, 153
injuries, databases of, 110
injury research database, 16
Inpatient Surgery site, 32
installation stage, 177

Institute for Quality and Efficiency in Health Care, 9
Institute of Medicine, 151, 153
institutionalized settings, study design, 152–153
Institutional Review Boards (IRBs), 167–168
instrumental activities of daily living (IADLs), 46
"Instrumental Variable Methods in Comparative Safety and Effectiveness Research," 88
instrumental variables, 88, 161–162
instruments, measurement. *See* measurement instruments; *specific instruments.*
Integrated Health Interview Series, 107
Integrated Public Use Microdata Series, 109
Integrated Public Use Microdata Series International, 109
Interactive Atlas of Heart Disease and Stroke, 136
International Clinical Trials Registry Platform (ICTRP), 24, 30, 170
International Compilation of Human Research Standards, 169
international health research, databases of, 110–111
International Household Survey Network, 111
International Human Development Indicators, 111
International Human Microbiome Consortium, 30
International Information System for the Agricultural Sciences and Technology (AGRIS), 15
International Network of Agencies for Health Technology Assessment, 9
International Society for Quality of Life Research, 49
International Society for Telemedicine & eHealth site, 27
International Standard Randomised Controlled Trial Register Number (ISRCTN), 169
interrupted time series design
    with comparators, 94–97
    in institutionalized settings, 153
Inter-University Consortium for Political and Social Research, 109
interventions, time issues, 145–146
Iowa State University, 36
IRBs (Institutional Review Boards), 167–168
irritable bowel syndrome, measuring patient-reported outcomes, 51
ISRCTN (International Standard Randomised Controlled Trial Register Number), 169

John M. Eisenberg Center for Clinical Decisions and Communications Science, 178
joint replacement, patient registry, 132

Kaiser Permanente clinical research, 102
Kelman, Charles, 186
Kids' Inpatient Database, 108

lifestyle factors in study participants, 128–129
life years, 52–53
likert scales, 44
literacy, measurement instruments, 52
location studied, effects on health
    built environment, 137–138
    County Health Rankings, 136
    drug use, variations in, 137
    emergency preparedness, 138
    GIS (Geographic Information Systems), 137–139
    Global Health Observational Map Gallery, 139
    health care workforce, 138
    HealthMap, 139
    HealthMap Vaccine Finder, 139
    health-related maps, 136
    health services, access to, 137
    Henry J. Kaiser Family Foundation, 136
    infectious disease modeling, 138
    Interactive Atlas of Heart Disease and Stroke, 136
    Medicaid coverage, 136
    overview, 135–136
    Robert Wood Johnson DataHub, 136
    targeting areas for screening, 138–139
    variations in medical services, 135–136
location studied, in study design
    comparators, structuring, 140
    geographical units, defining, 140
    outcomes, defining, 140
    patient-centered research, 140
logs, measurement instruments, 45
London, cholera epidemic, 88, 135
longitudinal databases, 102–103, 159
longitudinal studies
    databases of, 98
    description, 93–94
    emergency services, 154
    primary care settings, 151

MAPI Research Trust, 49–50
maps, health-related
    cancer, geographic distribution, 139
    cancer, mortality, 139
    Dartmouth Atlas of Health Care, 22, 135, 139
    Dartmouth Atlas of Health Care online, 138
    Global Health Observational Map Gallery, 139
    HealthMap Vaccine Finder, 139
    Henry J. Kaiser Family Foundation, 136
    Interactive Atlas of Heart Disease and Stroke, 136
    ZTCAs (Zip Code Tabulation Areas), 140
Markov models, 119, 158
masking, 64–65
Mayo Clinic, 179
McMaster University, 9, 171
means, evaluating outcomes, 55
measurement instruments
    ADLs (basic activities of daily living), 46
    administration, 52
    BADLs (basic activities of daily living), 46
    Barthel Index, 46
    burden, 52
    checklists, 44–45
    comparability, 52
    daily activities, 46–49
    diaries, 45
    disability, 53
    EUROQol, 46
    Functional Assessment of Chronic Illness Therapy, 47
    functioning, 46–49
    Health and Activities Limitations Index, 47
    health-related quality of life, 46–49
    Health Utilities Index, 46–47
    IADLs (instrumental activities of daily living), 46
    likert scales, 44
    literacy, 52
    logs, 45
    mental health settings, 48
    mobility, 46
    National Quality Measures Clearinghouse, 109
    objectives, 52
    Outcome Rating Scale, 48
    pain, 46–49
    personal care, 46
    pictorial response, 44
    Quality of Well-Being Scale, 47
    rating scales, 45
    reliability, 52
    respondent records, 45
    selecting, 51–52
    Session Rating Scale, 48
    SF-36 (Short Form Health Survey), 47
    target population, 52
    validity, 52
    validity of, 52
    VFQ-25 (Visual Functioning Questionnaire), 47
    vision and eye health, 47
    visual analog scales, 44
    See also checklists; questionnaires; surveys.

measurement instruments, for children
  chronic illnesses, 46
  developmental scales, 46
  Pediatric Quality of Life Inventory, 47–48
measurement instruments, patient-reported outcomes
  anxiety, 49
  asthma, 51
  cognition, 51
  Critical Path Institute, 50–51
  depression, 49, 51
  drug data, 50
  ePRO (Electronic Patient Reported Outcome) Consortium, 51
  fatigue, 49
  Genome-wide Association Studies, 51
  global health, 49
  International Society for Quality of Life Research, 49
  irritable bowel syndrome, 51
  MAPI Research Trust, 49–50
  National Quality Measure Clearinghouse, 51
  pain interference, 49
  Par-Qol (Participation and Quality of Life) project, 51
  Patient-Reported Outcome Consortium, 50–51
  for phenotypic research, 51
  PhenX Toolkit, 51
  PROLabels, 50
  PROMIS (Patient Reported Outcomes Measurement Information), 49
  PROMs (Patient Reported Outcome Measures), 49
  PROQOLID (Patient-Reported Outcome and Quality of Life Instruments Database), 50
  PROs (Patient Reported Outcomes), 49
  rheumatoid arthritis, 51
  sleep disturbance, 49
  social function, 49
  spinal cord injuries, rehabilitating, 51
  standardization efforts, 49
  types of instruments, 50
  users guide to implementing, 49
  See also outcomes, evaluation methods.
medians, evaluating outcomes, 55
Medical Care, 157
medical conditions
  questionnaires, 131
  in study participants, 131–132
medical devices
  classes, 25–26
  as comparators, 25–27
  examples of, 25
  FDA regulation, 25
  governmentally required studies, 26
  patient registry, 132
  registries, 27
Medical Literature Analysis and Retrieval System online (MEDLINE), 14, 16, 111–112
medical service variations, effects on health, 135–136
Medical Subject Headings (MeSH), 14
Medicare/Medicaid
  Centers for Medicare and Medicade Services database, 102
  Chronic Conditions Data Warehouse database, 103
  link to National Cancer Institute database, 103
  Medicaid coverage, effects on health, 136
medications
  as comparator, 23–25
  interactions, studying, 23–25
  See also drugs.
medications, safety
  regulatory agencies, 23
  studying, 23–25
  See also FDA (Food and Drug Administration).
Medicines and Healthcare Products Regulatory Agency, 23
MEDLINE (Medical Literature Analysis and Retrieval System online), 14, 16, 111–112
Medline Plus, 180
mental health services
  bibliographic databases, 15
  Substance Abuse & Mental Health Services Administration, 179
  See also psychotherapy.
mental health settings, measurement instruments, 48
MeSH (Medical Subject Headings), 14
meta-analysis
  cumulative, 116–117
  definition, 111
  forest plots, 116–117
  general procedures, 113–116
  heterogeneity, 118
  influence assessment, 118
  MOOSE (Meta-Analysis of Observational Studies in Epidemiology), 172
  online resources, 111–112
  PRISMA (Preferred Reporting Items for Systematic Reviews and Meta-Analyses), 171–172
  Proteus effect, 118
  relevant features, 116–118
  See also systematic reviews.

Meta-Analysis of Observational Studies in Epidemiology (MOOSE), 172
Metagenomics of the Human Intestinal Tract, 30
methodology register, 14
microbiome sites, 30
microorganisms, as therapy, 30
microsimulation, health policy studies, 158
Microsoft Academic Search, 16
microsumulation, 119–120
Mid-Atlantic Twin Registry, 132
Milbank Quarterly, 157
Millennium Cohort Study, 99
Millennium Development Goals Indicators, 111
MISCAN (MIcrosimulation for Screening Analysis), 119
mobility. *See* exercise and mobility.
Monte Carlo simulation, 119, 158
MOOSE (Meta-Analysis of Observational Studies in Epidemiology), 172
mortality data, databases of, 110
mortality rates
  by disease, 53
  evaluating outcomes, 53
  outcome evaluation, 53
mortality risk
  by age in population, 141
  patterns of, 141
multilingual translation searches, 18
multivariable adjustment, large databases, 161
mutations, 122

National Archive of Computerized Data on Aging, 108
National Asbestos Exposure Register, 132
National Cancer Institute (NCI). *See* NCI (National Cancer Institute).
National Center for Biotechnology, 178
National Center for Health Statistics
  Data Linkage Activities, 102
  health policy studies, 158
National Children's Study, 99
National Health and Nutrition Examination Survey (NHANES), 35, 108
National Health Interview Survey, 107
National Health System economic evaluation, 14
National Implementation Research Network, 176–177
National Institute for Health and Clinical Excellence (NICE), 9, 18, 173
National Institute for Occupational Safety and Health, 110
National Institutes of Health (NIH). *See* NIH (National Institutes of Health).
national insurance records, databases of, 102
National Library of Medicine, 180

National Physicians Alliance, 19–20
National Quality Measures Clearinghouse, 51, 109
National Registry of Evidence-based Programs and Practices (NREPP), 179
National Sample Survey of Registered Nurses, 109
National Surgical Quality Improvement Program, 31
National Technical Information Services, 112
Nationwide Emergency Department Sample, 108
Nationwide Inpatient Sample, 32, 108
NAT (Nutrition Analysis Tool), 36
natural cohorts, 99–100
natural experiments, 88
NCI (National Cancer Institute)
  ASA24 Automated Self-administered 24-hour Recall site, 36
  Diet History Questionnaire, 35–36
  geographic distribution of cancer, 139
  link to Medicare data, 103
  questionnaires on exercise and mobility, 37
  Risk Factor Monitoring and Methods Branch, 35–36
Netherland Information Network of General Practice, 98
Netherlands National Trial Register, 169–170
New England Journal of Medicine, 185
NHANES (National Health and Nutrition Examination Survey), 35, 108
NICE (National Institute for Health and Clinical Excellence), 9, 18, 173
NIH (National Institutes of Health)
  Health Care Systems Research Collaboratory, 75
  Health Information, 180
  PROMIS (Patient Reported Outcomes Measurement Information), 49
NNH (Number Needed to Harm), 58
NNT (Number Needed to Treat), 58–59
N-of-1 trials
  crossover effects, 81
  multiple outcomes, 81
  overview, 80–81
  precision and personalized medicine, 123
  washout periods, 81
  within-person design, 81
nonhuman entities, as comparator, 41
noninfectious diseases, databases of, 110
noninferiority trials, 84–85
nonrandomized trials
  description, 87–88
  emergency services, 154
  GRACE (Good Research for Comparative Effectiveness), 174

nonrandomized trials (*Cont.*)
   institutionalized settings, 152
   primary care settings, 151
   TREND (Transparent Reporting of Evaluations Nonrandomized Designs), 174
NREPP (National Registry of Evidence-based Programs and Practices), 179
null hypothesis, 12
Number Needed to Harm (NNH), 58
Number Needed to Treat (NNT), 58–59
nurses
   CINAHL (Cumulative Index to Nursing and Allied Health Literature), 112
   National Sample Survey of Registered Nurses, 109
   Nurse's Health Study, 99
Nurse's Health Study, 99
nursing and allied professions, database, 15
nursing facilities, designing studies for, 152–153
nutrition
   children, 110
   databases of, 15, 110
   infants, 110
   USDA site, 180
   women, 110
   See also diet and food.
Nutrition Analysis Tool (NAT), 36

Obamacare. *See* Patient Protection and Affordable Care Act.
observation, study design, 60
observational studies
   designing, 89–91
   MOOSE (Meta-Analysis of Observational Studies in Epidemiology), 172
   STROBE (Strengthening the Reporting of Observational Studies in Epidemiology), 174
obstetrics, dietary research, 35
odds, evaluating outcomes, 55
odds ratios, evaluating outcomes, 55–56
older adults, sample biases, 24
Online Label Repository, 23
online resources. *See* databases; search engines; *specific resources*.
oophorectomy, case study, 1
Open Grey, 112
organ studies. *See* biologics.
organ transplants
   human organs to humans, 29
   nonhuman organs to humans, 28
   xenotransplantation studies. *See* biologics.
original research studies, databases of, 111–112
Ottawa Hospital Research Institute, 180

Outcome Rating Scale, 48
outcomes
   categories, 43–44
   defining, 140
   evaluating, time issues, 142–145
   healthy lifespan, 52–53
   life years, 52–53
   predicting, 184
   primary, 53
   secondary, 53
   See also measurement instruments, patient-reported outcomes.
outcomes, evaluation methods
   absolute risk difference, 56
   Bayesian inference, 58–59
   confidence intervals, 57–58
   contrasting groups, 55
   difference, medical definition, 56
   differences between two measures, 55
   estimates of effect, 55
   means, 55
   medians, 55
   mortality rates, 53
   NNH (Number Needed to Harm), 58
   NNT (Number Needed to Treat), 58–59
   odds, 55
   odds ratios, 55–56
   overview, 53
   percentages, 54
   placebo groups, 56
   probabilities, 55
   proportions, 53
   P-value, 58
   random error, testing for, 58
   rate ratios, 55–56
   rates, 53
   rates of disease incidence, 53
   ratios of two measures, 55
   relative risk, 55–57
   risk differences, 56–57
   risk ratios, 55–56
   variability, assessing, 57–58
   See also measurement instruments, patient-reported outcomes.
outcomes, patient-reported
   measurement categories, 44–45. *See also* measurement instruments, patient-reported outcomes.
   overview, 44
Ovid search engine, 16
Oxford Centre for Evidence-Based Medicine, 9

pain, measurement instruments, 46–49
pain interference, measuring patient-reported outcomes, 49

pain measurement, time issues, 142
panel studies, designing, 100–102, 158
Panel Study of Income Dynamics, 101
parallel arms, 63
Par-Qol (Participation and Quality of Life) project, 51
participants in trials and studies. *See* study participants.
Participation and Quality of Life (Par-Qol) project, 51
Partners in Information Access for the Public Health Workforce, 108
patient-centered outcomes research. *See* comparative effectiveness research.
Patient-Centered Outcomes Research Institute (PCORI), 13–14
patient-centered research, 140
Patient Health Questionnaire depression module 9 (PHQ9), 45
Patient Protection and Affordable Care Act, 40
patient registries
    asbestos exposure, 132
    Australian Society of Cardiac Surgeons, 132
    Canadian Joint Replacement Registry, 132
    cohorts with common experiences, 133
    Danish Twin Registry, 132
    disease prevention, 132
    environmental health, 132
    European Cardiac Surgical Registry, 132
    FDA National Medical Device Registry, 132
    FDA Unique Device Identification System, 132
    medical devices, 132
    Mid-Atlantic Twin Registry, 132
    National Asbestos Exposure Register, 132
    radiation exposure, 132
    as research resource, 133–134
    Society of Thoracic Surgeons National Database, 132
    surgical procedures, 132
    Swedish Twin Registry, 132
    toxin exposure, 132
    UNC Health Registry, 132
    See also databases.
Patient-Reported Outcome and Quality of Life Instruments Database (PROQOLID), 50
Patient-Reported Outcome Consortium, 50–51
Patient Reported Outcome Measures (PROMs), 49
patient-reported outcomes
    bibliographic databases, 50
    measurement categories, 44–45. *See also* measurement instruments, patient-reported outcomes.
    overview, 44

Patient Reported Outcomes Measurement Information System (PROMIS), 49, 142
Patient Reported Outcomes (PROs), 49
Patient Safety Indicators, 98
Patient Safety Network, 98
PCORI (Patient-Centered Outcomes Research Institute), 13–14
Pediatric Quality of Life Inventory, 47–48
pediatrics, dietary research, 35
peer reviewed literature database, 15
PennState Online Data Archive for Population Studies (SodaPop), 109
percentages, evaluating outcomes, 54
perfect studies, designing, 165
period prevalence, 142
personal care, measurement instruments, 46
personalized medicine, 121–124
personal privacy, 169
pets, as comparator, 41
pharmacologic studies database, 14
phases of clinical drug trials, 23–24, 83
phenotypes, 122
phenotypic research
    measuring patient-reported outcomes, 51
    questionnaire for, 51
PhenX Toolkit, 51
PHI (Protected Health Information), 169
PHQ9 (Patient Health Questionnaire depression module 9), 45
physical activity. *See* exercise and mobility.
physical traits, 122
physicians
    average time of visits, 146
    British Doctors Study, 99
    characteristics, 109
    National Physicians Alliance, 19–20
Physiotherapy Evidence Database, 15
PICO (Population, Intervention, Comparison, Outcome), 11
pictorial response, measurement instruments, 44
placebos
    as comparators, 21–22
    evaluating outcomes, 56
    in trials, 64
plasmid therapy, 31
PLOS Medicine site, 39
POHEM (Population Health Model), 119–120
point-of-care testing, 148
point prevalence, 142–143
Population, Intervention, Comparison, Outcome (PICO), 11
population data, databases of, 110
practice-based evidence studies, designing, 100
pragmatic randomized control trials, 124
pragmatic trials, 72

precision medicine, 121–124
PRECIS (Pragmatic-Explanatory Continuum Indicator Summary), 72, 164
preference trials
 comprehensive cohort trial design, 86–87
 overview, 86
 randomization, 86–87
 Wennberg's design, 86
 Zelen's design, 87
pregnancy, dietary research, 35
pregnant women, in cohort studies, 99
prescription drugs. *See* drugs; medications.
Primary Care Service Areas, 109
primary care settings, study design, 149–152
primary outcomes, 53
primary prevention, 32
priorities, set by funding, 13–14
priorities for study design, 151
PRISMA (Preferred Reporting Items for Systematic Reviews and Meta-Analyses), 171–172
probabilities, evaluating outcomes, 55
probability value. *See P-*value.
prodromal period, 143
PROLabels, 50
PROMIS (Patient Reported Outcomes Measurement Information System), 49, 142
PROMs (Patient Reported Outcome Measures), 49
propensity analyses, large databases, 161
propensity score matching, 125
proportions, evaluating outcomes, 53
PROQOLID (Patient-Reported Outcome and Quality of Life Instruments Database), 50
PROs (Patient Reported Outcomes), 49
prospective cohort studies, 98
prospective trials, 63
Protected Health Information (PHI), 169
Proteus effect, 118
psychology
 bibliographic databases, 112
 database, 15
psychotherapy
 cognitive behavioral therapy, 38
 "Comparative Efficacy of Seven Psychotherapeutic Interventions for Patients with Depression...," 39
 as comparators, 38–39
 comparing approaches, 38–39
 Seeking Safety therapy, 38
 treating depression, 39
 See also mental health services.
PsycINFO
 bibliographic databases, 112
 description, 15
 searching, 16

public health data, databases of, 102, 108–111
Public-Use Data files and Documentation, 102
PubMed
 Clinical Queries, 154
 large databases, 159
 MEDLINE access, 16
PubMed Central
 biomedical literature, 18
 pragmatic randomized control trials, 124
 propensity score matching, 125
 type 1 diabetes, 17
 Web site, 16
P-value, 58

QUADAS (Quality Assessment of Diagnostic Accuracy Studies), 175
Quality of Well-Being Scale, 47
quasi-experimental studies, 87–88
questionnaires
 CDC Behavioral Risk Factor Surveillance System, 131
 Diet History Questionnaire, 35–36
 exercise and mobility, 37
 on exercise and mobility, 37
 family medical history, 131–132
 food frequency, 35
 Functional Assessment of Chronic Illness Therapy, 47
 Genome-wide Association Studies, 51
 medical conditions, 131
 National Health Interview Survey, 131
 online inspection tool, 51
 for phenotypic research, 51
 PhenX Toolkit, 51
 VFQ-25 (Visual Functioning Questionnaire), 47
 See also checklists; measurement instruments.
questions for research. *See* research questions.

race
 classifications, 127
 in study participants, 127–129
radiation exposure, patient registry, 132
random error, testing for, 58
randomization
 adaptive trials, 74
 controlled trial designs, 33
 preference trials, 86–87
 screening tests, 33
 See also trial design, randomization.
randomized trials
 checklist for reporting and publishing, 172–173
 design aid, 164
 selecting a study design, 164

randomized trials, adaptive trials
    fixed-size randomized trials, 74–75
    sequential randomized controlled trials, 75
    SMART (sequential multiple assignment randomized trial), 75
randomized trials, cluster trials
    example, 76
    overview, 76
    REDUCE MRSA trial, 76
    sequential enrollment, 77
    stepped wedge design, 76–78
randomized trials, with comparators
    description, 62–66
    emergency services, 154
    institutionalized settings, 152
    primary care settings, 150–151
random numbers, source of, 68–69
random permuted blocks, 70
ranked approach to selecting a study design, 162–163
rate ratios, evaluating outcomes, 55–56
rates, evaluating outcomes, 53
rating scales, 45
ratios of two measures, evaluating outcomes, 55
red blood cell transfusions, 185
REDUCE MRSA trial, 76
RefPRO, 50
registering trials, 24, 169–170
registries
    CENTRAL (Cochrane Central Register of Controlled Trials), 24, 112
    of controlled trials, 14, 169–170
    databases of, 103
    ISRCTN (International Standard Randomised Controlled Trial Register Number), 169
    methodology, 14
    National Asbestos Exposure Register, 132
    Netherlands National Trial Register, 169–170
    See also patient registries; *specific registries.*
relative risk, evaluating outcomes, 55–57
reliability
    measurement instruments, 52
    surveys, 107
RePEc (Research Papers in Economics), 15
reporting randomized trials, checklists, 172–173
ResDAC (Research Data Assistance Center), 103
research questions
    common questions asked, 5–6
    null hypothesis, 12
    scientific hypotheses, 12
    testing hypotheses, 12
research questions, formulating
    overview, 10–13

PCORI (Patient-Centered Outcomes Research Institute), 13–14
PICO (Population, Intervention, Comparison, Outcome) elements, 11
priorities, set by funding, 13–14
searching the literature, 14–18
standards for, 13–14
TRIP database, 11
Research Randomizer, 72
research studies. *See* studies.
respondent records, measurement instruments, 45
responses. *See* outcomes.
results. *See* outcomes.
ReThink Health, 120
retrospective cohort studies, 98
rheumatoid arthritis, measuring patient-reported outcomes, 51
risk, decision modeling, 119–120
risk differences, evaluating outcomes, 56–57
Risk Factor Monitoring and Methods Branch, 35–36
risk ratios, evaluating outcomes, 55–56
Robert Wood Johnson DataHub, 136
Robert Wood Johnson Foundation, 158
run-in period, 63–64

Safe Surgery Saves Lives program, 31
SafetyLit, 16
sample biases
    children, 24
    individuals with multiple diseases, 24
    older adults, 24
    women, 24
School Meals, 110
SciELO (Scientific Electronic Library Online), 16
Science Accelerator, 18
scientific hypotheses, 12
scientific literature, database, 15
scientific method, study design, 60
scientific observation, trial design, 89
scientific research, search engine, 18
Scirus search engine, 16
Scopus, 15
screening tests
    as comparators, 32–33
    definition, 32
    designing, 155–156, 157
    "Evaluating Test Strategies for Colorectal Cancer Screening…," 120
    list of, 33
    MISCAN (MIcrosimulation for Screening Analysis), 119
    primary prevention, 32
    randomized controlled trial designs, 33

screening tests (*Cont.*)
  secondary prevention, 32
  targeting areas for, 138–139
  tertiary prevention, 32–33
  US Preventive Services Task Force site, 33
search engines
  BASE (Bielefeld Academic Search Engine), 16, 17
  Bioinformatic Harvester, 18
  biomedical literature, 18
  biomedical original research articles, 16
  care transitions, 17
  CiteSeer, 16
  Department of Energy, 18
  Directory of Open Access Journals, 16
  Embase access, 16
  Europe PubMed Central, 17
  filtering results, 18
  genetic studies, 18
  Google Scholar, 16
  HubMed, 17
  information science, 16
  MEDLINE access, 16
  Microsoft Academic Search, 16
  multilingual translation searches, 18
  NICE (National Institute for Health and Clinical Excellence), 18
  Ovid, 16
  PsycINFO access, 16
  PubMed, 17
  PubMed Central, 16, 17, 18
  Science Accelerator, 18
  scientific research, 18
  Scirus, 16
  type 1 diabetes, 17
  WorldWideScience.org, 18
  See also databases; *specific search engines.*
searching the literature, 14–18
  See also databases; search engines.
secondary outcomes, 53
secondary prevention, 32
Seeking Safety therapy, 38
SEER (Surveillance, Epidemiology, and End Results) program, 98, 103
selection bias, large databases, 161
self-controlled case series, 91–93
sepsis, case study, 1
sequential multiple assignment randomized trial (SMART), 75
sequential randomized controlled trials, 75
Session Rating Scale, 48
sex, in study participants, 126–127
SF-36 (Short Form Health Survey), 47
"Shared Decision Making: A Model for Clinical Practice," 6

shoes, as comparator, 41
Short Form Health Survey (SF-36), 47
side effects, 25
skilled nursing facilities, designing studies for, 152–153
sleep disturbance, measuring patient-reported outcomes, 49
SMART (sequential multiple assignment randomized trial), 75
smokers, as study participants, 129–130
Smoking & Tobacco Use Surveys, 130
Snow, John, 88, 135
social aspects of health and disease, database, 16
social function, measuring patient-reported outcomes, 49
social science
  CESSDA (Council of European Social Science Data Archives), 110
  Social Science Research Network, 16
Social Science Research Network, 16
social support, as comparator, 38–39
Society of Thoracic Surgeons National Database, patient registry, 132
SodaPop (PennState Online Data Archive for Population Studies), 109
Solomon Four Group Design, 85–86
spinal cord injuries, measuring patient-reported outcomes, 51
SPIRIT (Standard Protocol Items: Recommendations for Interventional Trials), 173–174
split-body trials, 82–83
SQUIRE (Standards for Quality Improvement Reporting Excellence), 175
stages of evidence implementation, 176–177
Standards for Systematic Reviews of Comparative Effectiveness Research, 112
STARD (Standards for the Reporting of Diagnostic Accuracy Studies), 175
State Ambulatory Surgery Databases, 108
statins, decision aid for, 179
statistics
  hospitals, 97
  Injury Statistics Query and Reporting System, 97
  National Center for Health Statistics, 102, 158
  National Center for Health Statistics Data Linkage Activities, 102
  WISQARS (Web-Based Injury Statistics Query and Reporting System), 109
stem cell therapy, 30
stepped wedge trial design, 76–78
stratified random sampling, 70–71

STROBE (Strengthening the Reporting of Observational Studies in Epidemiology), 174
stroke, 136
studies of specific therapies
    common variables. *See* comparators.
    comparison groups, 20
    efficacy *vs.* effectiveness, 20–21
    evaluating outcomes, 55–59
    lack of, 2
    placebos, 21–22
    relative effectiveness, 58–59
    watch and wait, 22
    watchful waiting, 22
    See also clinical drug trials; outcomes.
study design
    case-control studies, 103–105
    cohort studies, 97–100
    common questions asked, 5–6. *See also* research questions, formulating.
    design elements, 61–62
    disease detection, 155–156
    emergency services, 153–154
    experimentation, 60
    health policies, 157–158
    home health services, 155
    hypothesis generation. *See* case-control studies.
    institutionalized settings, 152–153
    location, choosing, 135–140
    meta-analysis, 111–117
    observation, 60
    observational studies, 89–91
    panel studies, 100–102, 158
    participants, choosing. *See* study participants.
    personalized medicine studies, 104
    practice-based evidence studies, 100
    primary care settings, 149–152
    priorities, 151
    rare condition studies, 104
    scientific method, 60
    screening tests, 155–156, 157
    systematic reviews, 111–118
    trend studies, 96–97. *See also* interrupted time series design.
    twin studies, 104–106
    See also time issues; trial design.
study design, selecting a design
    contrast approach, 162
    gap method, 163–164
    for perfect studies, 165
    for randomized trials, 164
    ranked approach, 162–163
    upshot model, 163

study participants
    consent forms, 169
    ethical principles for treatment, 167–169
    genotypes, 122
    human subjects oversight, 167–169
    IRBs (Institutional Review Boards), 167–168
    most important characteristics, 126
    patient registries, 132–134
    personalized medicine, 121–124
    personal privacy, 169
    phenotypes, 122
    physical traits, 122
    precision medicine, 121–124
    propensity score matching, 125
    selecting, time issues, 145
study participants, describing
    age, 126
    alcohol intake, 129
    ethnicity, 127–129
    health-relevant lifestyle factors, 128–129
    medical conditions, 131–132
    overview, 124–126
    physical activity, 130–131
    race, 127–129
    sex, 126–127
    tobacco use, 129–130
Substance Abuse & Mental Health Services Administration, 179
Supplemental Nutrition Assistance Program, 110
surgical procedures
    Cochrane Summaries site, 32
    as comparators, 31–32
    Inpatient Surgery site, 32
    National Surgical Quality Improvement Program, 31
    Nationwide Inpatient Sample, 32
    patient registry, 132
    procedures in hospital settings, 32
    Safe Surgery Saves Lives program, 31
    World Health Organization Surgical Safety Checklist, 31
Surveillance, Epidemiology, and End Results (SEER) program, 98, 103
surveys
    Aging Integrated Database, 108
    American FactFinder, 107
    CDC Smoking & Tobacco Use Surveys, 130
    CDC Surveys and Data Collection Systems, 108
    demographic information, gathering, 107
    designing, 106–111
    examples, 107
    health-related data, 108–111
    Integrated Health Interview Series, 107
    National Archive of Computerized Data on Aging, 108

surveys (Cont.)
    National Health Interview Survey, 107, 131
    NHANES (National Health and Nutrition Examination Survey), 108
    overview, 106–107
    reliability, 107
    SF-36 (Short Form Health Survey), 47
    tobacco use, 130
    validity, 107
    See also measurement instruments; specific surveys.
Surveys and Data Collection Systems, 108
Swedish Twin Registry, 132
symptoms, checklists of, 45
systematic reviews
    AMSTAR (Assessment of Multiple Systematic Reviews), 175
    definition, 111
    general procedures, 113–116
    online resources, 111–112
    PRISMA (Preferred Reporting Items for Systematic Reviews and Meta-Analyses), 171–172
    study design, 111–118
    See also meta-analysis.
systematic reviews database, 14

target population, measurement instruments, 52
technology, time issues, 147–148
tertiary prevention, 32–33
testing hypotheses, 12
test subjects. See study participants.
TheNNT.com site, 58
Therapeutic Goods Administration
    medical device registries, 27
    responsibilities, 23
theses, databases of, 112
thrombocytosis, case study, 1
time issues
    average time of doctor visits, 146
    breast cancer, 143–144
    in clinical research, 146–147
    evaluating outcomes, 142–145
    hospital length of stay, 146–147
    implementing interventions, 145–146
    increased use of technology, 147–148
    infection process, 143
    in-hospital mortality, 147
    overview, 141
    pain measurement, 142
    period prevalence, 142
    point-of-care testing, 148
    point prevalence, 142–143
    selecting participants, 145
    in study design, 145–146
tissue studies. See biologics.

tobacco use in study participants, 129–130
"Toward Precision Medicine: Building a Knowledge Network for Biomedical Research and a New Taxonomy of Disease," 122
toxin exposure, patient registry, 132
toxin studies. See biologics.
training for researchers, 103
Transfusion Requirements in Critical Care (TRICC) trial, 185
transfusions. See blood transfusions.
translation searches, 18
trend studies, designing, 96–97
TREND (Transparent Reporting of Evaluations Nonrandomized Designs), 174
trial design
    allowing change during implementation. See adaptive trials.
    assigning by user preference. See preference trials.
    case-crossover design, 91–93
    clinical drug trials, 83
    comparing for equivalent outcomes. See equivalence trials; noninferiority trials.
    comparing measurement instruments. See Solomon Four Group Design.
    confounding factors, 66
    delayed start trials, 84
    dose response trials, 83–84
    drugs, in human trials. See clinical drug trials.
    effects of different doses. See dose response trials.
    equivalence trials, 84–85
    evaluating in real-world settings. See pragmatic trials.
    evaluating under ideal conditions. See explanatory trials.
    experimentation vs. observation, 89–91
    explanatory trials, 72
    factorial trials, 82
    Health Care Systems Research Collaboratory, 75
    instrumental variables, 88, 88
    interrupted time series with comparators, 94–97
    longitudinal designs, 93–94
    measuring effectiveness over time. See interrupted time series design; longitudinal studies.
    multiple in same study. See factorial trials.
    natural experiments, 88
    naturally occurring. See natural experiments.
    noninferiority trials, 84–85
    nonrandomized trials, 87–88
    overview, 60–61

pragmatic randomized control trials, 124
pragmatic trials, 72
PRECIS (Pragmatic-Explanatory Continuum Indicator Summary), 72
prospective trials, 63
quasi-experimental studies, 87–88
randomized trial, active comparators, 62–66
randomizing. *See* crossover trials.
scientific observation, 89
self as test subject. *See* case-crossover design; self-controlled case series.
self-controlled case series, 91–93
single subject. *See* case-crossover design; N-of-1 trials; self-controlled case series; split-body trials.
on a single test subject. *See* case-crossover design; within-person design.
Solomon Four Group Design, 85–86
split-body trials, 82–83
subjects with shared characteristics. *See* cohort studies.
symptomology, separating from disease progression. *See* delayed start trials.
without randomization. *See* nonrandomized trials; quasi-experimental studies.
See also study design.
trial design, adaptive trials
  CONSORT (Consolidated Standards of Reporting Trials), 75
  eligibility criteria, 73
  fixed sample size, 74–75
  fixed-size randomized trials, 74–75
  interim analysis showing beneficial effect, 74
  interim analysis showing lack of effect, 74
  overview, 73
  randomization, 74
  sequential randomized controlled trials, 75
  SMART (sequential multiple assignment randomized trial), 75
  study populations, 74
  unexpected outcomes, 73–74
trial design, cluster randomized trials
  example, 76
  overview, 76
  REDUCE MRSA trial, 76
  sequential enrollment, 77
  stepped wedge design, 76–78
trial design, crossover trials
  issues, 79–80
  overview, 78
  within-person design, 78
trial design, elements of
  blinding, 64–65
  concealed randomization, 65
  controls, 63
  masking, 64–65
  placebos, 64
  run-in period, 63–64
  See also arms.
trial design, N-of-1 trials
  crossover effects, 81
  multiple outcomes, 81
  overview, 80–81
  precision and personalized medicine, 123
  washout periods, 81
  within-person design, 81
trial design, preference trials
  comprehensive cohort trial design, 86–87
  overview, 86
  randomization, 86–87
  Wennberg's design, 86
  Zelen's design, 87
trial design, randomization
  blocking, 69–70, 71
  block size, determining, 70–71
  concealed randomization, 65
  conducting, 68–69
  equalizing groups, 69–70
  equalizing identical twins, 67
  practice site, 72
  preparing for, 67–68
  purpose of, 66
  random permuted blocks, 70
  Research Randomizer, 72
  source of random numbers, 68–69
  stratified random sampling, 70–71
trial design, types of comparisons
  between-person, 65
  cluster, 65–66
  within-person, 65
trial participants. *See* study participants.
trial protocols, checklists, 173–174
trials
  of drugs. *See* clinical drug trials.
  registering, 169–170
  See also studies.
TRICC (Transfusion Requirements in Critical Care) trial, 185
triggers for blood transfusions, 185
TRIP database, 11, 17
twin studies
  comparators, 105
  Danish Twin Registry, 132
  fraternal (dizygotic) *vs.* identical (monozygotic), 105
  genetic environmental influences, 105
  identical (monozygotic), equalizing, 67
  Mid-Atlantic Twin Registry, 132
  Swedish Twin Registry, 132
  targeting interventions, 105–106
type 1 diabetes, 10, 16, 17

UNC Health Registry, 132
United States Department of Agriculture (USDA). *See* USDA (United States Department of Agriculture).
University HealthSystem Consortium, 102
University hospital Medical Information Network Clinical Trial Registry, 169–170
University of Illinois, 36
University of Minnesota
    Integrated Health Interview Series, 107
    Nutrition Data System for Research, 36
University of Washington, 111
upshot model for selecting a study design, 163
URLs. *See specific web sites.*
Usability.gov, 180
US Agency for Healthcare Research and Quality, 178
USDA (United States Department of Agriculture)
    AGRICOLA, 15
    databases of food content, 36
    nutrition programs, 110, 180
US Department of Health and Human Services. *See* DHHS (Department of Health and Human Services).
US National Library of Medicine, 16
US Preventive Services Task Force, 9, 33
usual care, as comparator, 22–23

vaccines
    HealthMap Vaccine Finder, 139
    immunizations, databases of, 110
    See also biologics.
vaccine therapy, 29–30
validity
    construct, 52
    content, 52
    criterion, 52
    measurement instruments, 52
    surveys, 107
    types of, 52
variability, assessing, 57–58
variables. *See* comparators.
VFQ-25 (Visual Functioning Questionnaire), 47
violence data, databases of, 110
virus therapy, 31
vision and eye health
    cataract surgery, 186
    measurement instruments, 47
visual analog scales, 44

washout periods, N-of-1 trials, 81
watch and wait, 22
watchful waiting, 22
Watson, IBM computer, 160, 184
weather predictions, 141

Web-Based Injury Statistics Query and Reporting System (WISQARS), 109
Webby Awards, 180
Web of Science, 15
websites
    awards for, 180
    creating, 180
    See also specific sites.
Wennberg's design, 86
WHO (World Health Organization)
    Clinical Trails Registry Platform, 53
    disability, world report on, 53
    disease burden, measuring, 52–53
    eHealth, definition, 27–28
    European portal, 158
    Global Health Observatory, 110–111
    Global Observatory, 158
    good health, definition of, 43
    Health for All Database, 110
    ICTRP (International Clinical Trials Registry Platform), 170
    International Clinical Trials Registry Platform, 24
    Surgical Safety Checklist, 31
    templates of human consent forms, 169
    tobacco use surveys, 130
    world report on disability, 53
WISQARS (Web-Based Injury Statistics Query and Reporting System), 109
within-person design
    case-crossover design, 91–93
    crossover trials, 78
    description, 65
    N-of-1 trials, 81
    primary care settings, 151
    self-controlled case series, 91–93
    split-body trials, 82–83
women
    maternal health, 110–111
    nutrition, 110
    pregnant, in cohort studies, 99
    sample biases, 24
    Women, Infants, and Children program, 110
Women, Infants, and Children program, 110
Wonder, 109
workplace safety, 110
World Bank, 110
WorldCat, 15
World Medical Association, 169
world report on disability, 53
WorldWideScience.org search engine, 18

xenotransplantation studies. *See* biologics.

Zelen's design, 87

www.ingramcontent.com/pod-product-compliance
Ingram Content Group UK Ltd.
Pitfield, Milton Keynes, MK11 3LW, UK
UKHW021329180426
11947UKWH00017B/1528